MINISTRY TO OUTPATIENTS

GUIDES TO PASTORAL CARE SERIES

Ministry to Persons with AIDS:
A Family Systems Approach
by Robert J. Perelli

Ministry to Outpatients:
A New Challenge in Pastoral Care
by Herbert Anderson, Lawrence E. Holst,
and Ronald J. Sunderland

GUIDES TO PASTORAL CARE

G·P·C

MINISTRY TO OUTPATIENTS

A NEW CHALLENGE IN PASTORAL CARE

**HERBERT ANDERSON
LAWRENCE E. HOLST
RONALD H. SUNDERLAND**

Published in cooperation with
the College of Chaplains of the
American Protestant Health Association

AUGSBURG • MINNEAPOLIS

GUIDES TO PASTORAL CARE SERIES

Consulting Editors

Laurel Arthur Burton
Joan M. Hemenway
Arne Jessen

MINISTRY TO OUTPATIENTS
A New Challenge in Pastoral Care

Scripture quotations unless otherwise noted are from the Revised Standard Version of the Bible, copyright © 1946, 1952, and 1971 by the Division of Christian Education of the National Council of Churches.

Library of Congress Cataloging-in-Publication Data

Ministry to Outpatients : a new challenge in pastoral care / Herbert
  Anderson, Lawrence E. Holst, Ronald H. Sunderland.
      p.   cm. — (Guides to pastoral care series)
    Presentations made at the First National Conference on Outpatient
  Ministry held in Houston, Jan. 1988, cosponsored by the M. D.
  Anderson Cancer Center and the College of Chaplains of the American
  Protestant Health Association.
    Includes bibliographical references.
    ISBN 0-8066-2508-2 (alk. paper)
    1. Pastoral medicine.   2. Patients—Pastoral counseling of.
  3. Hospitals—Outpatient services.   4. Clinics—Psychological
  aspects.   I. Anderson, Herbert, 1936–   .   II. Holst, Lawrence E.
  III. Sunderland, Ronald, 1929–   .   IV. National Conference on
  Outpatient Ministry (1st: 1988: Houston, Tex.)   V. M. D. Anderson
  Cancer Center.   VI. American Protestant Health Association. College
  of Chaplains.   VII. Series.
  BV4335.M56   1990
  259'.4—dc20   90-21895
                                                              CIP

The paper used in this publication meets the minimum requirements of American National Standard for Information Sciences—Permanence of Paper for Printed Library Materials, ANSI Z329.48-1984.   ∞™

Manufactured in the U.S.A.   AF 9-2508

95   94   93   92   91   1   2   3   4   5   6   7   8   9   10

CONTENTS

5

FOREWORD

Growth in outpatient care is affecting health care delivery in much the same manner that supermarkets replaced the corner grocery a generation ago. Not only has what we *do* changed, but it has changed in a positive direction, for it is clear that the long-range impact of such change is serving the best interests of patients. Many factors are contributing to this radical change in health care delivery.

Ten years ago, few hospital administrators would state that outpatient facilities produced any income. Hospital administrators shunned clinics and hoped others would take care of that need because it did not add to the "bottom line." In another ten years, 25 percent of a hospital's income from all sources will come from ambulatory care.

Since 1970, the average length of hospital stay has been halved. Where once the national average was 13 days, it is now 6 days. In acute care hospitals, the average stay has been reduced from 17 days to 8. Across the United States, the average hospital occupancy rate in 1970 was 90 percent because utilizing beds was the preferred way of treating patients in all hospitals. Today the average occupancy rate throughout the nation is approximately 65 percent, and administrators and trustees are growing more comfortable with that. During the 1980s, hospital admissions were falling at a rate of one million every two years despite population growth, the rapid aging of the population, and the fact that the number of people needing hospitalization was growing.

While some people maintain that the reason for the trend toward outpatient care is an oversupply of physicians, this is not the case. The problem with respect to access to physicians is the maldistribution of doctors. There are too few in critically underserved areas like rural communities and inner cities; there are not too many.

Efforts to curtail health delivery costs also contributed to this trend. The responsibility for paying for hospital care moved from the individual to insurers, and then to other various forms of third-party payment. Employers began to assume a major portion of these costs, and the federal government became involved through Medicare and Medicaid. With rapidly escalating health care costs, agencies at every level began to institute cost-curtailment measures, hoping, for example, that market competition would play a large part.

New construction, termed "over-bedding," once was a common method of meeting hospital costs. It was justified by the conviction that more beds were needed because physicians could not provide quality care away from inpatient facilities. Now that trend has been reversed, due in part to new technologies resulting in improved surgical and medical protocols and delivery methods. It is the revolution in medical technology that has made the greatest impact on our ability to undertake many procedures in outpatient clinics that were previously restricted to inpatient facilities.

Changes in health care delivery began to appear even before pressures for cost curtailment were felt, due to emerging new medical technologies. For example, following passage of the National Cancer Act of 1971, cancer research in the United States began to receive serious support for the first time. By 1971, research funding from all sources—voluntary, federal, state, and private—amounted to only $271 million. By 1976, there had been a fourfold increase in funds for cancer research. As a result of the infusion of new federal research dollars, we have learned more about the causes of cancers and how to cure cancer than in all previous human history. The past 15 years have been the most productive period in both cancer medical research and practice. The benefits derived from this exploding volume of knowledge have played a major part in our ability to care for patients in outpatient clinics. It is readily acknowledged that this is in the best interests of patients in a far greater number of medical situations than previously was recognized or possible.

The task of a hospital is not only to heal patients whenever possible, but to help those patients achieve a life-style at least equal to, if not better than, that which preceded their hospitalization. We are seeing that vision realized for growing numbers of patients, yet in many ways we have failed to educate the public to accept the cured cancer patient. Subtle and not-so-subtle discrimination is still high. We are curing many cancer patients, somewhere in the range of 60 percent, but our task is not complete unless patients reintegrate into family life, are able to continue in their occupations, and play the fullest roles open to them as members of their communities. For many patients cancer care rendered in outpatient settings is a significant step in this direction.

There are many reasons for preferring outpatient cancer treatment when that is an option. First, in outpatient clinics, home-based hospices, and prevention and screening clinics offered at worksites and schools, we are seeing a different kind of attitude toward responsibility for completeness of care. Ambulatory cancer care is at least as good, if not better, with lower toxicity and better therapeutic results. For example, using new portable chemotherapy pumps, M. D. Anderson Cancer Center has treated nearly 12,000 patients on an ambulatory basis in preference to inpatient care. Packaged chemotherapy is refrigerated at home and a family member is trained to oversee the patient's long-line catheter. This procedure has resulted in cutting the cost to patients by two-thirds and that to the hospital by one-third.

One of the most important benefits is the quick return of patients to their home settings. This permits them to return to employment and reconstitute their lives, rather than lying in a hospital bed for weeks at a time. Patients may now be cared for with fuller family support, less disruption of family life, and maximization of family resources than was possible for chronically ill patients in the past.

The problem of psychological dependence in patients is another issue that is being affected by the trend toward outpatient care. Whether overt or subliminal, some patients are apt to feel: "I don't want to get too far from these walls, because therein lies my hope and strength." Patients with this mind-set have misplaced their faith. They begin to put too much confidence in the medical environment that surrounds them and fail to utilize all their personal strengths to overcome their illness.

The consequences of the burgeoning growth in outpatient care also affect the chaplain's ministry. As care has moved from the bedside to clinics, we have become aware that, for the patient and the staff, clinics are places that provide little privacy. Quick vignettes take the place of extended visits with chaplains. For example, there is less opportunity to minister to patients who undergo same-day admissions or day surgery, and then return home. As essays in this volume propose, perhaps the primary responsibility for pastoral and spiritual support for outpatients will rest with congregational clergy and members, and institutional pastoral staffs will need to serve in a supplementary capacity. Departments of pastoral care may then commit resources to orient clergy to our clinics and focus attention on our facilities to provide for clergy continuing education as our contribution to achieving the most effective reintegration of patients to their homes, communities, and congregations.

As these issues are clarified, and as long as we work together to identify and serve our patients' interests, visits to outpatient clinics will be much less traumatic. Patients' needs for developing their own spiritual strengths will not lessen. But because hospital staff will not be able to allocate the time with patients to assist them to develop and sustain these spiritual strengths during their brief time in the institution, there is an understandable concern on the part of chaplains that they may fail to serve ambulatory patients as well as they serve patients in the hospital. It was to facilitate discussion of these issues that M. D. Anderson Cancer Center supported the First National Conference on Outpatient Ministry held in Houston in January 1989 and the dissemination of those deliberations in this volume.

Changes in the health care delivery system are making a major impact upon consumers, health care institutions, and caregivers whose lives are devoted to patient care. Every hospital staff member and every department is faced with challenges arising from these changes. The revolution may be near its peak, but we still do not know what the future will bring. However, we will manage these changes, learn from them, and serve our patients more effectively if we remember that we are faced with opportunities, not with problems.

Charles A. LeMaistre, M.D.
President, The University of Texas
   M. D. Anderson Cancer Center
Houston, Texas

PREFACE

The trend toward outpatient care is altering the shape of medical practice and the way hospital administrations and the general public view health care delivery. As essays in this volume indicate, this trend is also altering the ministry of chaplains and pastors.

Pastoral care for people attending outpatient clinics is not new; the clinics have always been with us. But they have not received high priority as areas for ministry, having been eclipsed by inpatient responsibilities. The fundamental question is, Are there any substantial differences between the two areas of ministry? If so, the differences need to be clearly defined so that ministry can be shaped accordingly. There can be no doubt that ministry in outpatient clinics is not only valid but important. Why, then, has outpatient ministry been on the back burner for so long, and what must be done to turn up the heat? This volume is based on the presentations made at the First National Conference on Outpatient Ministry held in January 1988, cosponsored by M. D. Anderson Cancer Center and the College of Chaplains of the American Protestant Health Association. It was planned as a first step in widening the investigation into outpatient pastoral care in the hope that the concerns we raise will be taken up across the nation. The essays presented in this volume were prepared initially for presentation to the conference.

In chapter one Herbert Anderson addresses the pastoral dimensions of outpatient clinic ministry in the context of a reconsideration of the chaplain's role in health care institutions, the unique features of the clinic, and the certainty that the role of the chaplain will change as medical treatment changes. He maintains that any adaptation of ministry in the clinic setting must be rooted in the theology and traditions of the respective faith groups. He poses three questions: What are the special circumstances and needs of the growing outpatient population? What new strategies does clinic ministry evoke? What is the role of the chaplain in today's hospitals?

His lively depiction of the pressures upon clinic patients sets the stage for answers to these questions. Patients are under duress because of the waiting invariably imposed upon them, the new levels of responsibility patients must accept for their own treatment, and their vulnerability to disease and to an institution's treatment protocols. Each aspect of his presentation is couched in theological terms that bring new insight to the roles of the clinical chaplain and parish pastor as they minister to outpatients.

In chapter two Lawrence Holst examines the present state of health care in the United States and the likely effect of health care policies at all levels—local, state, and national—on pastoral ministry by the staffs of hospital departments of pastoral care. For example, pastoral caregivers may expect to be held more accountable for the quality of their work as institutions require monitoring of quality and measuring of outcomes. Holst proposes six strategies to assist pastoral care personnel to design and implement effective clinic ministry. He concludes with a statement of conviction that, in view of the crisis faced by health care generally and hospital chaplaincy in particular, the pressure is on chaplains to adapt to the new boundaries and limits that are shaping their world.

Chapter three distills the insights of four staff chaplains who work at the University of Texas M. D. Anderson Cancer Center. Virgil Fry shares the irritation he experienced when forced to wait in the clinic area himself, and reflects on the lessons chaplains may learn while observing and ministering to patients and their families who must wait in a sea of anxiety evoked by anticipation of the news and information they fear they will hear from physicians. Nathan Huang reflects on the discomfort that most chap-

lains experience when walking into a crowded clinic waiting area
and the strategy he has implemented to meet the demands created
by this setting. He illustrates his contribution with clinical episodes. Both Fry and Huang find the focus of ministry in the
chaplain's presence and openness to the needs of people.

Geri Opsahl addresses the needs of outpatients in the specialized setting of the outpatient or day-surgery clinic, where anxiety
common to any hospital care center is exacerbated by the anticipation of the surgical procedure for which the patient is scheduled. She suggests that pastoral care is, or ought to be, informed
by two models: external and internal. The former refers to the
physical and verbal actions of the chaplain; that is, being present
and serving as a channel of communication within the surgery
system. The latter model identifies the intrinsic roles of the chaplain, expressed in the form of sensitivity, intentionality, visibility,
and "readiness."

Sister Margaret Whooley reflects on her ministry, wondering
if she is able to take the risk involved, to evoke the potential in
outpatients so they become part of their own healing and to help
them in their spiritual searching. She emphasizes the importance
of healing relationships on all levels: individual, family, and institutional.

The final four chapters touch on additional topics related to
outpatients—clinic-parish connections, a ministry of openness,
ministry in community health centers, and ministry to people
with AIDS.

Ron Sunderland outlines the investigation undertaken by staff
chaplains at the M. D. Anderson Cancer Center, beginning with
their review of pastoral ministry in outpatient clinics prior to
1987 and the considerations that led to the decision to convene
the conference on outpatient ministry. He reviews the possibility
of working with the clergy and members of the congregations
from which the patients come to outpatient clinics. He discusses
the chaplains' growing awareness that they first need to explore
difficulties that may inhibit their own clinic ministries. Second,
he states that they need to establish clearer guidelines for clinic
ministry before incorporating training programs into their work
in the clinics. Nevertheless, Sunderland calls for a recognition
on the part of departments of pastoral care that the ministry

exercised by parish clergy and laity is essential to the pastoral care of outpatients. It is far more extensive than that which hospital staffs can offer outpatients; and he suggests a point of interface between a patient's congregation and the work of the pastoral care department.

Betty Adam describes the physical setting of the clinic waiting area and the moods it evokes. Like other staff members she anchors pastoral care in the attitude of openness that she believes is incumbent upon chaplains. She sets the foundation for this ministry of openness in a theological framework of God's openness to humankind. She urges pastoral caregivers to be open to moments that "transcend our finite perspective." Like Huang and Opsahl, Adam emphasizes that under the open model, chaplains learn to be both physically and spiritually present in the clinic as much as possible, particularly in the waiting areas where visibility is crucial. This presence may consist simply in introducing oneself to people. This requires a certain "boldness," for when there is no specific request for service from patient or staff, no list of patients on which to make check marks, no summons to here or there, "what remains is a sea of people and the spontaneous encounter that is its own fulfillment."

Lorna Miller describes another setting for outpatient ministry, community health centers. As a chaplain, she works with patients in the Harris County Hospital District, which serves the medically indigent people of Houston, Texas, and surrounding communities. The needs and situations vary widely. One outpatient may be an alcoholic woman who lived under bridges in Houston for three years but now is sober; another may be a teenage refugee from El Salvador. Miller recalls Matthew 25:40 (paraphrased), "Whenever you did it for one of my brothers or sisters *here,* you did it for me."

Mary Grace addresses the prophetic role of chaplains in relation to outpatient care for persons with AIDS. She looks at two large categories of difficulties these people face. One is the hospital's institutional nature that depersonalizes patient care, and the other is the often catastrophic intraphysic stresses that may lead to psychotic breaks. Grace emphasizes the importance of real community for persons with AIDS and tells what several churches in San Antonio have done to meet that need.

Ronald H. Sunderland

Chapter 1

PASTORAL REFLECTIONS ON OUTPATIENT CARE

Herbert Anderson

At the conclusion of the book he edited, *Hospital Ministry: The Role of the Chaplain Today,* Lawrence Holst suggested that chaplains need new visions and the will to pursue them.[1] Those new visions are a necessity because hospitals are changing. There will be fewer hospitals; treatment procedures will be more technical and specific; health care will be more narrowly defined, competitive, and entrepreneurial; and cost-effectiveness will be the criteria for treatment modalities. This essay addresses one particular change in hospital procedure: the increase in outpatient treatment and the decline in numbers of hospitalized patients. This change has wide-ranging consequences for the ministry of chaplains and parish pastors.

In order to understand the theological dimensions of outpatient care, it is necessary to reconsider the role of chaplains and pastors in the hospital and clinic. It will also be necessary to explore the unique features of the outpatient clinic context and the particular needs of the outpatient in order to determine an appropriate pastoral response. This consideration of the theological dimensions of outpatient care points to larger questions regarding the church's role in today's health care. The role of the chaplain in particular will change as medical treatment changes. The reasons for these changes need to be rooted in the church's mission as well as in the needs of the sick and suffering.

Outpatient care is many-faceted. It includes the networks of care for people living with AIDS and the growing practice of parish-based health care staffed by nurses and other professionals. It includes home births and home-based care of those who are mentally handicapped or emotionally troubled. Outpatient treatment also includes hospice care at home, infertility clinics and abortion clinics, genetic counseling clinics, consultation of the elderly, same-day surgery care, rehabilitation programs, and ongoing treatment of the seriously or chronically ill.

Because this essay was presented at the first conference on pastoral ministry and outpatient care, it is appropriate that we begin with more questions than conclusions. We might conclude that the outpatient treatment context is more like the doctor's office than the hospital and therefore is not a necessary context for pastoral care unless we were to propose that there be chaplains in doctors' clinics. Or we might conclude that the spiritual resources of the church's care must be available for all people who are ill, outpatients as well as inpatients. Or we may conclude that some outpatient contexts more than others present personal and spiritual concerns that warrant the presence of a chaplain or a pastor. My intent is to explore some criteria for examining the church's response to outpatient care.

This is crucial not only because methods of medical treatment are changing. It is important for us to reappraise continually the allocation of the church's resources. Protestant churches do not yet face the kind of shortage of pastoral personnel that is approaching crisis proportions in the Roman Catholic Church. But there is a curious and potentially serious crisis emerging in Protestant churches as well. Although there is no shortage of interest in full-time ministry in or on behalf of the church, more and more people would rather be in some form of specialized ministry than parish ministry. Therefore local congregations with declining membership are being asked to support more and more expressions of ministry in the public arena. The church simply cannot do all of the good and even necessary things it feels called to do. For that reason the allocation of the church's increasingly limited resources will require careful evaluation of the many situations of human need that call for pastoral response. Outpatient treatment contexts are only one of many genuine situations that call for Christian ministry to point to the presence of God and be an advocate for human need.

There are, it seems to me, three kinds of questions that will help us examine the pastoral dimensions of outpatient care. (1) What are the special circumstances and needs of the growing outpatient population? (2) If it is true that context shapes our pastoral response, what new pastoral strategies does the outpatient context bring forth? What are the limits to the privilege of pastoral initiative? How will the more public nature of outpatient care change the promotion of psychological intimacy that has characterized the relationship between patients and chaplains or pastors for several decades? (3) What is the role of the chaplain in the hospital today? To what extent is a pastoral care presence in outpatient treatment a logical extension of the role of hospital chaplain? How is it different?

The Special Needs of Outpatients

Although our pastoral response is never solely determined by the needs and circumstances of the people whom we seek to serve, one of the marks of the modern pastoral ministry of care is that it takes human need seriously. Because the church is attentive to each individual's experience, it is important that we begin by asking about the special needs of those in outpatient care. Their needs are diverse because outpatient care is highly specialized and varied. The needs of a couple at an infertility clinic are not the same as those of patients at a diagnostic center for problems of aging, or of those undergoing the rigors of chemotherapy, or of those in outpatient treatment for same-day surgery. Despite such diverse needs, there are some common aspects of the outpatient experience. I would suggest these: (1) the waiting may not be as long but it can be more intense; (2) outpatients are more responsible for their treatment processes; and (3) medical treatment is a part of their ordinary routine.

1. *Waiting.*   Outpatients spend a lot of time waiting. My friend Erma who runs the newsstand near my home said it simply: "People do a lot of waiting in waiting rooms." Sitting in a chair

reading a back issue of *Redbook* feels more like waiting than lying in a hospital bed dozing or watching TV does—even though both are in anticipation of the same or similar medical procedures. Outpatient waiting may not be as long as the waiting of a hospitalized patient, but it can be more stressful. It is an intensification of the experience of waiting that is familiar to us all.

We live in a society that does not encourage waiting. We honk our horns at the driver ahead if he or she delays ten seconds after the light turns green. We may choose not to buy something rather than wait in line. We shoot people who cut in ahead of us on the Los Angeles freeway. We are angry when our plane is delayed or a friend is late for dinner. We think about waiting in terms of powerlessness, helplessness, and passivity. And we think of being active and in control of the use of time as power. Our ordinary experiences of waiting do not prepare us for the experience of being seriously ill.

In one of his homilies, Paul Tillich observed that "waiting means not having and having at the same time."[2] We wait for what we do not have, for what we do not know, for what is yet to occur, for someone who is yet to come—and that is not easy.

A friend of mine who was abandoned by her mother at an early age observed, "That experience established in me the habit of waiting and expectation that makes any present moment most significant for what it does not contain." Waiting means not possessing. It is an experience of emptiness. And so we wait for God because we do not possess God. We wait for death because we do not possess death. We wait for health because we do not possess health.

Waiting is not having, but it is also having. The fact that we wait for something shows that in some way we already possess it. If we wait in hope and patience, the power of that for which we wait is already effective within us. Tillich remarked, "He who waits passionately is already an active power himself, the greatest power of transformation in personal and historical life. *We are stronger when we wait than when we possess.*"[3] (italics mine) That is a powerful reminder about the dangers of idolatry, about presuming to possess God or health, or presuming that finally we can control life.

What the person suffering from a serious or life-threatening illness knows better than the rest of us is that "we are much stronger when we wait than when we possess." I suspect that the outpatient also knows about having and not having at the same time. If I am able to drive myself to the clinic for treatment, I am well enough. When I am waiting for the light to turn green, I am reasonably sure that the people in the car next to me cannot see that I am an outpatient. My friends and colleagues at work may even describe me as the "picture of health." But when I sit in the outpatient waiting room, waiting for treatment, I am aware that health is not something I possess. And at that moment, if Tillich was correct, I am stronger. I am stronger in that moment of waiting because I know that I have nothing. And once I know that I have nothing I can be anything, and in that realization is wonderful freedom and splendid strength.

I am indebted to an English writer, W. H. Vanstone, for the idea that waiting is more than passivity. In a book entitled *The Stature of Waiting*, Vanstone concluded that working and waiting are both part of the nature of God and human nature at its best.[4] We are no less blessed when we wait upon the world than when we are working and achieving in it.

Almost every waiting room is a room full of waiting. In that waiting—in pain, fear, loneliness, or terror—we discover this deeper truth: that waiting is every bit as important as achieving. In the radical receptivity of our waiting, we can understand, appreciate, and welcome in ways that are not possible when we are busy making, achieving, and possessing. It is our waiting that discloses life in its heights and depths. Waiting discloses the secret of the world's power of meaning: to welcome, to appreciate, to understand the world that comes to those who wait. We are stronger when we wait than when we possess. That is something outpatients know very well.

2. Being responsible. The second characteristic of the outpatient experience has to do with patient responsibility. There is greater expectation that patients will take responsibility for their treatment. This perspective is promoted through a myriad of guides to self-help during treatment. In a sense it is a corrective to the infantilizing tendency that has often been identified with hospitalization. The structure, routines, and rules of in-hospital treatment promote medical authority and patient dependency. Patients do not always know the treatment plan. Some would rather not know. Others are too sick. They need to be taken care of because they are incapable of taking care of themselves. They are acted upon because they are incapable of acting themselves. They are dependent upon the care of medical personnel in order to devote their own limited energies to the task of getting well.

The circumstances of outpatients are quite different. They are very likely fully engaged in the tasks of living—earning a living, caring for children, looking after parents, talking to neighbors—in addition to the task of getting well. Outpatients can be responsible participants in the healing process in a variety of ways: one patient must remember not to eat or drink for 24 hours before the medical procedure; another needs to remember to take a regimen of medication before and after the outpatient treatment; a third will monitor the effect of medication on patterns of eating and drinking in order not to undermine the healing process. Like those who suffer from chronic illness, outpatients need to become experts on their own bodies. In that sense, they are responsible partners in the treatment process.

A friend of mine had a mastectomy almost two years ago. Since then she has taken charge of her body. She became well informed about the disease process and was a model outpatient throughout chemotherapy. She was able to cope by anticipating the negative side effects of the medication. With the support of other women who have had breast cancer, she has radically altered her patterns of eating and drinking. All of these changes in her life have given her a new sense of what it is to be a responsible self. She chose not to be a victim of her illness even if her life might eventually be shortened because of it. Instead, she chose to be a responsible participant in the healing process.

This emphasis on responsible partnership in the treatment process is very important for individuals living with AIDS. The term, people with AIDS (PWA), is designed to remove any sense that someone with AIDS is either victim of the disease or a patient with a terminal sickness. Every effort is made to be well informed about the disease process and to assume responsibility for the treatment process. The emphasis is on *living* with AIDS rather than dying from AIDS. A person with AIDS is determined to live until he or she dies. Although some denial may be operative in the failure to come to terms with death, the emphasis on life highlights the point that outpatient care requires a greater responsibility on the part of the patient to be a participant in the treatment process.

At least two major changes must occur if patients are to take more responsibility in the treatment process. First, the medical world needs to be demystified enough so that when we are patients, we are willing to insist on the information that is essential for responsible management of our illnesses or our treatment processes. Some physicians recognize that knowledgeable patients make better patients, others do not. But because of the mystique we attach to physicians, we hesitate asking them much. It is likely that they are willing to teach us more than we want to know. There is something lost in the way many people order their world if physicians are perceived to be gods. However, what is gained is far greater than what is lost. Because being knowledgeable about one's illness is so crucial for outpatient care, patient education must be a standard part of the treatment protocol.

The second attitudinal shift that needs to occur in order to increase responsible outpatient participation is a religious one. Our theological anthropologies have emphasized dependency more than partnership in relationship to God. To insure that the process of salvation is wholly God's doing, some traditions have de-emphasized human agency in general. H. Richard Niebuhr's classic consideration of *The Responsible Self* continues to provide a useful construct for thinking about human agency.[5] We are responding and responsible selves in the midst of community. The self is always a social self. And our selfhood, in the midst of community, is defined by our ability to respond to the actions of others upon us. To paraphrase Niebuhr, we are, as outpatients, responsible selves in the management and treatment of illness. This participation in our healing is an extension of understanding human beings as responsible partners with God.

This emphasis on the responsible care of ourselves has also generated a popular emphasis on preventive health. The health club business and our society's general preoccupation with health have contributed to a new tyranny: we can stay healthy if we eat right, modulate stress, and exercise properly. The "ideology of health," which reduces the ideals of self-knowledge and self-mastery to a regimen of diet and exercise, amounts to the "medicalization of American individualism." Health becomes a "dawn-to-dusk regimen, with plenty of bedside reading, health books having replaced philosophy or religious books as guides to the good life."[6] George Will is right to caution about confusing health maintenance with the conquest of mortality. Sometimes the connection between responsible behavior and good health is obvious. However, more often than not it is a mystery. As Montaigne wrote, "You do not die of being sick, you die of being alive." Deciding to live carefully or to be a responsible partner in outpatient care is important but it does not eliminate finitude. Tillich was correct: we need to accept suffering with courage as an element of finitude and affirm finitude in spite of the suffering that accompanies it.[7]

3. *Treatment as a daily routine.* The third common theme in outpatient care is the overlap between the medical world and the ordinary world. My treatment may be part of a daily routine that also includes work and play. That possibility has the potential for normalizing sickness and medical treatment. The impact of the outpatient experience on our self-understanding may be to eliminate any dichotomy between being sick and being human.

Some years ago James Ashbrook wrote a splendid essay, "The Impact of the Hospital Situation in Our Understanding of God and Man,"[8] in which he suggested that being hospitalized is an experience of brokenness. The wholeness of life has been disrupted. Life has become separated and estranged from its dynamic wholeness. That sense of brokenness is not only physical; it is emotional and spiritual as well. The hospitalized sick, according to Ashbrook, are separated and maybe even estranged from themselves, from significant communities of friends and family, and from God. The brokenness we know in a hospital setting encompasses all of life. Brokenness may not be the dominant metaphor used to describe the human plight today, but it is still an accurate picture of what people feel who are sick enough to be hospitalized. It is not just that some body parts are in need of repair; they are broken.

The outpatient experience is less clear. My hunch is that vulnerability is a more suitable metaphor for the outpatient experience than brokenness. You have not completely broken down if you are well enough to drive yourself to the clinic or if you do not need a wheelchair to leave the treatment center. The constant awareness of struggles between life and death in the hospital is muted slightly in the outpatient setting by signs of health and the patient's mobility. People think that if you are up and around, you cannot be that sick. And yet, the wound is not healed over, fatigue is pervasive, or the outpatient may leave the clinic wearing a Foley catheter or a somewhat disguised shunt for dialysis. All of those are unmistakable signs of vulnerability.

There is also a more pervasive sense of vulnerability because outpatient care softens the boundaries between who is sick and who is well. My mother always used to say if I was sick enough to stay home from school, I had to stay in bed. She was a nurse and she knew about hospital rules. However, according to outpatient practice a person might be sick enough to need treatment (that is, stay home from school) and still be mobile. Outpatient care challenges us to rethink definitions of health that emphasize the absence of disease and to favor instead a more functional understanding of health.

The rethinking of our understanding of health is a theological as well as medical task because it calls us to reconsider our assumptions about human nature. According to the anthropology that undergirded in-hospital care, we assume that most of us are healthy most of the time but sometimes we get sick. If, however, the experience of outpatient care is the basis for developing our understanding of human nature, we might say that sickness is the norm and that most of the time most of us function pretty well nonetheless. If I have had a particularly difficult session with my psychiatrist, I often forget to take off my purple tag that identifies me as an outpatient. So there I am, pedaling my bicycle all over Hyde Park and broadcasting my status as an outpatient. I am embarrassed by the image, but when I cut away my defenses I think it is right. It is like the general confession in the old Anglican Common Book of Prayer that would require us to declare at least once a week that there is no health in us. We are all finite creatures. Outpatients know better what most of us seek to hide by layers of character armor—that we are all very vulnerable. And very, very fragile. In that sense we are all outpatients.

If we continue to use the old way of thinking in outpatient treatment, people are likely to forget that they are still sick after they leave the clinic. If we continue to believe that being out of the hospital means we are not really sick, we are in danger of forgetting that we have limited reserves because of our treatment or our lingering sickness. If we are responsible for our treatment, then we are also responsible for monitoring the expenditure of energy.

My friend Connie went in for laparoscopic laser procedure recently. Her husband Dave took her to the clinic on his way to work and promised to pick her up later. She waited two hours for a procedure that took 45 minutes. Then she waited another two hours for Dave to pick her up, but he forgot. Finally Connie took a cab home only to discover that Dave had invited his friend Richard home from work. Richard, who appeared to have more sensitivity than her husband, took one look at her fatigue and found an excuse to leave. Dave is not the most sensitive man in the world but neither is he a first-class cad. I suggest that he is still working out of an old anthropology: If you are mobile, you are not really sick.

There are problems about ongoing care when people leave the hospital sicker than was true in the past. Current outpatient treatment presumes that those people have a home to go to, with someone to care for them. That is a questionable assumption because more and more people live alone. And it presumes well-developed therapeutic and social services that people can utilize effectively in their homes. Outpatient treatment also presumes well-established networks that will be able to coordinate a variety of services that may be necessary to maintain daily living. The chronic nature of outpatient treatment will require structures of supportive maintenance in which the church may play a significant role.

There are other dynamics common to the outpatient experience. Waiting for test results always generates anxiety. Being seriously ill is a terrifying thing. Outpatient care provides a limited safety net around those fears. Even though the infections that an individual is likely to pick up at home are more ordinary and therefore more easily treatable than the germs produced in hospitals, many people would rather be in a hospital when they are sick. Although being hospitalized is often an isolating experience, to live alone and be chronically ill can be even more isolating. We must continue to explore both ordinary and unusual aspects of outpatient care in order to determine the church's ministry of pastoral care within this mode of medical treatment. Expressions of pastoral care on behalf of the church are always shaped by the particular needs of the sick and suffering to whom we minister. In what ways might a ministry of pastoral care in outpatient treatment take a different form because of the particular needs of that context?

The Pastoral Response
to Outpatient Needs

I suggest three aspects of the practice of pastoral care that may be slightly different in an outpatient ministry. The first is pastoral initiative. What is the rationale for pastoral initiative in a clinical context? Are there any limits to pastoral initiative outside the chaplain-patient relationship or a pastoral relationship within a religious community? The second is advocacy. Outpatient care, even more than in-hospital treatment, calls for the pastoral caregiver to be an advocate on behalf of people and their needs. The third aspect of the church's ministry in an outpatient setting I call supportive maintenance. Of all the types of outpatient care, treatment of the chronically ill is one of the most emotionally debilitating for the patients and their families. The church has a particular opportunity to provide support for the chronically ill and their families.

1. *Pastoral initiative.* I agree with Lawrence Holst that initiative is essential for effective pastoral care.[9] However, I would describe it more as a privilege than a right. It is not so much inherent in the office of pastor, as Holst suggests, as it is in the pastoral relationships that are established and maintained within religious communities. It is a privilege of the covenant rather than a right of the office. The pastor's or chaplain's access to

hospitalized patients and their families is a complicated mixture of this pastoral privilege and the medical right of access.

Both the urbanization of society and the professionalization of pastoral ministry have contributed to a decline in the exercise of the privilege of pastoral initiative. People in cities live behind several locked doors to protect themselves from unwelcome or unexpected visitors. Twenty-five years ago, when I got into my car to make parish calls in Citrus Heights, California, I could expect to find people at home and willing to receive an unexpected guest. Today, that is an exception. When we are home, even our closest friends are unlikely to drop in unannounced. Today the wise pastor will make an appointment in order to practice pastoral initiative.

Our freedom to take initiative with patients and their families is a sacred trust. It is easier to think about exercising that sacred trust within a hospital setting than in an outpatient context. For example, with whom would one begin to take initiative in the public space of a waiting room: the person seated nearest the door, the one person who looks familiar, the one who smiles when our eyes meet, or the outpatient with an empty chair next to him or her? Some outpatients will occupy a separate room for a while, but primarily for medically related purposes. The chaplain may have a space to which he or she might like to withdraw with an outpatient for a more private conversation, but pastoral initiative may be limited by an already full schedule of prior appointments.

The outpatient context raises a number of questions about pastoral initiative. How will pastoral conversations with outpatients be different if they occur in public settings? What kind of demonstration of pastoral availability is appropriate in an outpatient waiting room that might prepare the way for pastoral initiative? If the chaplain is an integral part of the treatment team, should the chaplain make home visits if the patient already has a pastor who visits regularly? If the person in rehabilitative therapy does not belong to a congregation, on what theological grounds would we be granted the privilege of initiative? Further, does pastoral initiative extend to the nearby motel where people in extensive outpatient treatment are staying while away from home?

In an unpublished paper, "Toward a Theology of Visitation," Kenneth R. Mitchell suggested two purposes for pastoral visitation to which I would add a third.[10] First, he said, we are living out the model of the Good Shepherd whom we encounter in the Gospels. By means of pastoral visitation we know those who are in our care and are known by them; we understand which ones are strong and which ones are weak, and thereby foster a relationship of trust. It is possible for us to care for them and to lead them only if we know them and they know us well.

Second, when we call on people, we personalize the gospel. That is, we provide the opportunity for one human being's story, one family's story, in all its particularity to come into contact with *The Story*. I believe Mitchell is correct. Unless the minister comes to know something of the uniqueness of each individual story, our efforts to bring this person into vital awareness of the good news of Jesus Christ will not make much sense.

I add a third dimension of pastoral visitation that is more subtle but no less essential. When we visit people in their hospital rooms and certainly when we visit them in their homes, we are their guests. Our parishioners will try to "lead us out," to get us to talk about ourselves, about the life of the church, about what happened to dear old Mrs. Anderegg. They will assume that we are the one with important gifts to give. If we are faithful in our pastoral visitation, something quite different happens. We invite the hosts to talk about *their* lives and we listen in a pastoral way. As we do that, we become the hosts, and our parishioners become the guests: guests, if you will, in their own home or hospital room.

It is a pastoral visit when we replicate God's becoming a guest among us in order to be our host. In our pastoral work we do not quite become hosts but rather stand-ins for the Host. We do host-like things in the Host's name. We make people comfortable in talking about themselves, we offer them the warmth of caring and listening, we may even take the lead in a celebration or ritual of sorts—all host-like activities.

To be a guest is the gospel experience. Our ministries of hospitality are an extension of God's coming among us to be our Host. In that sense, our pastoral visitation in the homes of parishioners or in the rooms of patients is a gospel paradigm. It requires some effort to imagine how that ministry of hospitality might be effected in relationship to outpatient treatment. The waiting rooms where they wait and where we meet are very public places. A chaplain will need to be very clever in finding ways to transform the space by someone's chair into a hospitable context. Such a gracious encounter may become increasingly essential if, as has been suggested, outpatient treatment comes to resemble a body shop where restoration work is done according to the predetermined payment. But people are more than gallbladders or malfunctioning kidneys. They have names and stories. It is the privilege of pastoral initiative to be the Host as we invite people to tell their stories.

2. *Advocacy.* In a sense the second aspect of the church's ministry in an outpatient context, advocacy, is an extension of pastoral initiative. The church needs to be prepared to function as an advocate for people for the following and many more reasons: (a) Because outpatient care has the potential to disregard the whole person in favor of precise treatment of specific body parts; (b) because outpatient care in its specificity is likely to continue to multiply specializations; (c) because the multiplication of specializations will make it difficult for people to find their way to the medical help they need without some guidance; (d) because increasingly effective medical technology will continue to generate complex ethical decisions for people to make; and (e) because cost effectiveness may prompt institutions to overlook the human dimension of care.

That advocacy role would certainly include prophetic speech. Although chaplains have worked hard to be regarded as full members of the health care team, they would not be there if their identity and values were not anchored outside the hospital and health care world. *It is a paradox of pastoral ministry in the medical context that pastors and chaplains belong precisely because they are outsiders.* It is their "outsiderness" that gives them the perspective they need to be prophetic. They bring a different vision. And therefore what they see is different. Because the value of the person transcends the values of health and because we know that finally we die because we are alive, not because we are sick, we see beyond medical technology.

Although specific caregivers in certain settings must speak a prophetic word in response to flagrant violations of human personhood or to the development of procedures that diminish rather than enhance the human spirit or to allowing cost effectiveness alone to set policy, the prophetic role in relation to health care institutions must be an agenda for the church as a whole. The concerns evoked by the development of outpatient treatment move us beyond pastoral care concerns to a broader health care agenda.

On the streets of any major city in America we see all too vividly the consequence of deinstitutionalization in mental health care. I do not mean to suggest a direct parallel between the policies that emptied our mental hospitals onto city streets and the growing practice to limit or avoid medical hospitalization. But we need to be sure that when people are sent home to heal, they have a home to go to and someone to care for them. A recent issue of *Chicago Reporter* carried these headlines: "Strapped Inner-city Hospitals Dump Patients to Avoid Red Ink." The extent to which we have allowed capital gain to be the determining factor in the care of the sick and suffering is one sign of the moral bankruptcy of our society.

Advocacy, understood very broadly, will also take the form of ethical guidance on a more personal level. Many outpatient programs have a diagnostic focus. The purpose is to gather accurate information in order to make an informed assessment so that the most responsible maintenance or treatment procedure might be determined. Gerontological outpatient clinics are therefore designed to help a family assess whether it is wise for grandmother to continue to live alone. Once the data is gathered, difficult, emotionally charged ethical decisions need to be made. Most of us need assistance in making ethical choices that are complicated by emotional bonds.

A former student of mine, Frank D. Seydel, now with the Division of Genetics of Georgetown University Medical Center, wrote to me recently. He directs the prenatal diagnostic laboratory, does genetic counseling with patients, and codirects a program of education for pastoral care in genetics. Genetic disease and birth defects pose a unique set of concerns for affected individuals and their families for which clergy, he said, are generally ill-prepared. The rapid expansion in the diagnosis and treatment of birth defects and genetic disorders has generated a new set of ethical questions that occur at the intersection of pastoral care, bioethics, and genetic counseling.

We could gather a long and perhaps overwhelming list of outpatient settings in which people must make complex ethical decisions without the leisure of lying in a hospital bed and perhaps without the support of family and friends. The questions will not go away because our technology continues to progress. More and more people will have to decide whether they must do what they can do. As with prophetic advocacy, issues related to ethical guidance and outpatient care transcend the limits of pastoral care. It is an agenda for the church.

The third expression of a ministry of advocacy is necessitated by the growing complexity of medical care. University of Chicago hospitals have approximately 120 different outpatient units. I have been confused on a couple of occasions when I had to select where I needed to go from the myriad of medical options available. Although I am well educated, reasonably intelligent, and even somewhat familiar with hospitals, I was still confused. It was like letting my fingers do the walking through the yellow pages. It works just fine as long as you know exactly what you want and the correct category under which to find it. But for many people, finding their way through the outpatient medical maze is so overwhelming that they do not seek the treatment that would be restorative.

If you are in the hospital, treatment procedures will be set in motion without the patient deciding what needs to be done next. There is less anxiety because the patient makes few choices. You do not need to know much. Since you may not get to choose, it is less frustrating not to know too much. If, on the other hand, the setting for care is the outpatient clinic, you need to know more because you are more in charge of your treatment. People who are anxious and confused about what they must do next will need a guide or an advocate, someone who knows them and knows the system well enough to be an advocate for the help they need. That kind of advocacy is needed *before* arriving at the hospital or outpatient clinic.

The new parish nurse programs that are springing up are addressing this genuine need for advocacy in outpatient care.[11] (In this program, a congregation provides a wholistic ministry for its members by adding a nurse to its staff to serve as a minister of health on a part-time or full-time basis. The parish nurse serves as a health consultant, educator, patient advocate, trainer of volunteers, and organizer of support groups.)

The parish nurse fulfills an especially useful function in support of persons needing outpatient care, particularly for the urban poor and disenfranchised. In a sense, the advocacy ministry of the parish nurse may be more beneficial than that of a chaplain because the nurse is with the people at the grass roots. The chaplain is sometimes as difficult to find as the eye clinic. And the parish may be the best context for advocacy both on behalf of persons and the treatment process.

Outpatient care introduces new questions about the role of advocacy in pastoral care. As outpatients become more active participants in the treatment process, I suggest a more active role for the clergy as well. And that advocacy role is enhanced by the awareness that the church stands with an outpatient outside the medical institution. The fact that chaplains are outsiders on the health team becomes an increasingly central paradox for the church's ministry of pastoral care in an outpatient context.

3. *Supportive maintenance.* I have already suggested that outpatient care is a multidimensional reality. Some of the care is acute and some is routine. However, even routine prenatal screening can be frightening for a woman over 35. Some outpatient care is remedial and the prospects for recovery are very good. Other outpatient care is rehabilitative and recovery may take longer and be uncomfortable. Some outpatient treatment such as interventional radiology is palliative and the expectation of recovery is only temporary. Some outpatient treatment allows people who are chronically ill to live reasonably full lives.

I suspect that there is no aspect of outpatient treatment that is a greater challenge to the church's ministry than the care of the chronically ill. Those who are chronically mentally ill are only one group, albeit a complex one, in this population. Chronically ill people live with the vulnerability of pain and the pain of vulnerability, and they teach us all about finitude. For most chronically ill persons and their families, the fact that they continue to live is the victory.

In a book entitled *The Illness Narratives: Suffering, Healing, and the Human Condition*, Dr. Arthur Kleinman of Harvard Medical School tells of his encounter with Paddy Esposito when Kleinman was a medical resident. He had been assigned to an inpatient rehabilitation unit that specialized in the care of quadriplegic and paraplegic adolescents. One of his responsibilities was to organize and run a small weekly group therapy session for six to eight paralyzed adolescents. On one afternoon the group decided to discuss suicide. After listening for a while to a rather gloomy conversation about suicide as an acceptable option for the severely impaired, Dr. Kleinman dealt with his own anxiety by rehearsing why suicide was not helpful and even cowardly and how with the passage of time they could come to accept their condition as something they would be able to live with. All of a sudden, Kleinman reports, a 16-year-old who had fractured his lower spine in a diving accident shouted an obscenity at him and then said, "You don't have to live this way the rest of your life. What do you know about what it's like to be in our condition? How dare you tell us what to do? If you were like us, you'd want to die too."[12]

Anger is a common emotion for the outpatients who are chronically ill and for the families and friends who care for them. Kleinman offers a method of care for the chronically ill that emphasizes empathic listening, the translation of medical knowledge in response to the patient's need to know about risk and vulnerability, and a therapeutic process of re-moralization that seeks to help the chronically ill person and his or her family express their grief in order to explore the meanings of the illness. His emphasis on negotiation and collaboration between physician and patient is another illustration of responsibility as a major theme in outpatient care. He suggests that the real challenge is for the physician to engage in negotiation with the patient as a colleague and collaborator. Of all the tradecraft of the physician, nothing more effectively empowers the patient.[13]

The church, one would hope, is potentially a very effective resource of care for the chronically ill and their families. The religious community understands itself as a community of sufferers. The mark of a religious community that embodies the love of God is its capacity to embrace suffering as a part of the human condition. It teaches that people are never less than human when they are sick or suffering. It cares for the chronically ill, offers companionship to the dying, and consoles those who grieve significant losses and injustices in life, even when it is not possible to cure what is broken or change what is wrong.

Healing is what we do as a religious community. It is also what we hope for. But because of the tenacity of evil in the world and the pervasiveness of ill-health, healing in this life is never complete. Therefore, from a theological perspective, it is possible that we all are "outpatients" who need one another to endure. We welcome the chronically ill into our midst as an exaggerated expression of us all because we are never more human than when we are sick or when we suffer.

The local religious community is ideally suited to provide supportive maintenance that will enhance medical outpatient care. If a religious community fulfills its highest ideals, it will be a place that holds people who are in pain. It is a place that loves the chronically cranky without needing to be loved in return. It is a place that does not overlook the need to care for those for whom cure is not likely. It is a place where the privilege of pastoral initiative allows access to people who have isolated themselves and been isolated by their illnesses. The mobilization of networks of care for persons with AIDS is one illustration of the kind of supportive maintenance possible for those who are chronically ill.

Chaplains in Outpatient Clinics?

I began this essay by asking what the church's response of pastoral caregivers to outpatient care should be. In a sense, we have been at work on that question all along. But still the question remains. What is the church's ministry of pastoral care in an outpatient setting, and by what means might that care be effected? That is similar to, but a little different from, asking about the role of the chaplain in the hospital. In what ways might we conclude that pastoral care in an outpatient setting is a logical extension of chaplaincy? And in what ways is it not? The emerging dominance of outpatient treatment sharpens the question of the relation between chaplaincy and the local congregation or religious community.

There is no doubt that people in outpatient treatment could benefit from the kind of care that we call pastoral. Some of the fears characteristic of hospitalized patients may be intensified in outpatient care. It is an ambiguous good that the loss of personal boundaries or the isolation from one's regular community is likely to be less in outpatient care. We will increasingly be responsible participants in the treatment process. Many people welcome the end of ignorance and passivity in relation to their own treatment process. For others, who welcome being taken care of when they are sick, becoming more responsible is terrifying. The needs of an outpatient population are great.

The church's role in outpatient treatment will be determined not only by need but by our understanding of the role of the chaplain in health care in general and hospital-based medical treatment in particular. If the chaplain's role is understood as a bridge between two worlds, outpatient care raises new questions because the boundaries between those two worlds have diminished. The outpatient does not withdraw from the world of computers and Pampers to be treated medically. If the outpatient has a sense of inbetweenness, it is temporary but still very intense. He or she will be back at work in the afternoon or tomorrow or at least sleep in his or her own bed. There is much temporary inbetweenness in human life today that could profit from signs of God's presence. Day-care centers, senior citizens centers, and mental health treatment centers are all places of inbetweenness where people spend time each day. By what criteria do we decide which situation needs the ministry of care most? Although it will continue to be essential to minister to people in situations of inbetweenness, it is possible that the base from which we begin will need to be the parish in order to maximize our freedom to respond where the need is the greatest.

If one regards chaplaincy as a public ministry, as Don Browning does, then one would probably decide that chaplaincy is an essential part of outpatient care because it supports the values of health. Browning contends that "God's general concern with creation, its fulfillment and its health, constitute the theological grounds of the Christian chaplain's public ministry in a pluralistic patient population. The hospital chaplain performs this public ministry in the service of health. The chaplain does not speak about the meaning of salvation or attempt to induce a religious experience except in order to detect elements of a patient's beliefs that might be working against the possibility of getting well."[14] From this perspective there is no inherent reason not to extend the ministry of chaplaincy into outpatient care. From this perspective, the limits are likely to be more pragmatic than religious.

If one regards the ministry of care in a health care setting as derivative in origin and representational in purpose, then the development of outpatient care raises new questions about the chaplain's role. One of the benefits of outpatient treatment (but one that is also accompanied by liabilities) is that people are not isolated from their primary communities of support. To be sure, not everyone has a supportive family or church or company of friends or colleagues. The number of people who live alone and isolated is increasing. But we can assume that many people who are treated as outpatients will, at the end of that treatment, return to a familiar and more or less supportive context.

The role of the chaplain in an outpatient clinic is an issue of authority as well as identity. As I have already suggested, we are always outsiders in the health care context and must be in order to retain our critical voice. That is the central paradox of chaplaincy. We are on the health care team precisely because our values, authority, and identity are grounded outside the health care context. And if our purpose for being a presence in health care institutions is to function on behalf of religious communities from which patients have been isolated, then outpatient care (in which that isolation is temporary) raises new questions about the church's direct role in this new treatment procedure.

In addition to these new questions, the emergence of outpatient care is likely to foster new modalities of caregiving on behalf of the church with people in this situation of inbetweenness: the parish nurse, parish networks of care that function in part as health advocates, or maybe simply outpatient companions who are willing to accompany someone through the medical maze. In the parish we will need to be hospitable to self-help groups that are organized around a common experience of illness. Such new modalities of ministry will take seriously the communities in which we live and the social systems that enhance or diminish the possibilities of human health and wholeness. Such new ministries will be responsive to the social embeddedness of illness *and* health. We do not get sick alone and we do not get better by ourselves. Such new modalities of care will be governed by an anthropology that recognizes that the boundaries between who is sick and who is well are less clear than in the past.

The needs for pastoral care in an outpatient setting are far greater and more diverse than the resources available. It is not possible to have a chaplain or pastor present wherever outpatient treatment is conducted. The outpatient clinic is not the only needy context. There are so many places where a sign of God's presence is needed. Some criteria other than need will be necessary to allocate the church's resources for the ministry of care. For instance, it could be decided, for the sake of the future of the human community, that day-care centers more than outpatient clinics need the ministry of care that chaplains are trained to provide. Because the questions that are raised are serious and far-reaching, the development of outpatient treatment programs is likely to precipitate a critical moment in the modern history of chaplaincy.

Notes

1. Lawrence E. Holst, ed., *Hospital Ministry: The Role of the Chaplain Today* (New York: Crossroad, 1987), 68–78.

2. Paul Tillich, *The Shaking of the Foundations* (New York: Charles Scribner's Sons, 1948).

3. Ibid.

4. W. H. Vanstone, *The Stature of Waiting* (London: Darton, Longman & Todd, 1982).

5. H. Richard Niebuhr, *The Responsible Self* (New York: Harper & Row, 1963). To be human is to be a responding creature and our responding is shaped by our interpretation of the meaning of action upon us; cf. 47–68 particularly.

6. George F. Will, "Grandmother Was Right," *Newsweek*, 16 January 1989, 68.

7. Paul Tillich, *Systematic Theology,* vol. 2 (Chicago: The University of Chicago Press, 1957), 70.

8. James Ashbrook, "The Impact of the Hospital Situation on Our Understanding of God and Man," in *Religion and Medicine,* ed. David Belgum (Ames: Iowa State University Press, 1967), 61–80.

9. Holst, *Hospital Ministry,* 68–78.

10. Kenneth R. Mitchell, "Toward a Theology of Visitation," unpublished essay.

11. Granger E. Westberg, *The Parish Nurse* (Minneapolis: Augsburg, 1990).

12. Arthur Kleinman, M.D., *The Illness Narratives: Suffering, Healing and the Human Condition* (New York: Basic Books, 1988), 139.

13. Ibid., 227–51.

14. Don S. Browning, "The Chaplaincy as Public Ministry," *Second Opinion,* vol. 1 (1986): 67–75.

Chapter 2

GETTING PASTORAL CARE BEYOND THE HOSPITAL'S WALLS

Lawrence E. Holst

A few decades ago some of us among the clergy made an important decision that has impacted our future: We chose to align ourselves with hospitals, seeking inclusion into the medical establishment. As a result, many of us find ourselves on hospital, not church, payrolls, directly accountable more to hospital administrators than to bishops.

It has worked well for the most part. Hospitals made a claim upon us, held us accountable, and provided vital financial and structural support. As hospitals flourished, so did chaplaincy.

And in the 1960s, 1970s, and early 1980s hospitals did flourish. Health care was under a reimbursement system that was favorable to growth, hospitals being the major beneficiary. It was a retrospective, cost-plus, fee-for-service, reimbursement system. The more services hospitals generated, the more revenues they received. It was a system that highlighted access and services—especially inpatient services.

As those services expanded, so did the number of professional people needed to provide them, including chaplains. Health care became the nation's second largest employer (after education), employing one of 14 working Americans, with an annual payroll of $60 billion. We were in heaven and did not know it!

But costs skyrocketed until we reached a point in the U.S. when health care was costing about $650 billion annually, or 11.5 percent of our gross national product. Joseph Califano reported that Chrysler had to sell 70,000 vehicles in 1985 just to pay its $400 million health care costs.[1] Today American business reputedly spends more on health insurance premiums (38 percent of its pretax profits) than it pays dividends to its shareholders. It has been predicted that health insurance premiums would climb 18–20 percent in 1989. Health care is doubling the nation's 3–4 percent inflation rate. Unchecked, it was feared that our nation's annual health bill could reach a trillion dollars in the 1990s. Industry, labor unions, the government, private insurers, and consumers began to scream in unison: "Enough!"

It appears that America has reached a point where hospitals are providing more health care services than the public can, or wants to, afford. Society, like individuals, must choose how and where it will spend its money. Currently, we spend as much on recreation as we do for health care. Desires in life are infinite; but resources are finite.

We are at a point where we can no longer balance access, quality, and affordability. Something, somewhere, somehow in that equation has to give. As Daniel Callahan reminds us: If we have *access* and *affordability*, we will have to change our notions of quality; if we have maximum *quality* and hold down *costs*, we will have to change our ideas about *equity;* if we have equal *access* and high quality, we will have to dedicate many more dollars to health care.[2] It is as simple and as complicated as that. Consequently, our consumer-patients and third-party payers are determined to be more prudent buyers of health care. Shopping for health care and advertising to increase one's share of the market are commonplace.

Change is everywhere. We are probably too close to the situation to appreciate that we are in the midst of a revolution in the delivery of medical services. That revolution has to do largely, but not only, with reimbursement. Money! A radically new reimbursement system for Medicare patients is upon us that is based on diagnosis-related groups (DRGs), a prospective, fee-for-illness system that is forcing hospitals to be more cost-effective, quality conscious, and competitive. (If you carefully contrast that with the more familiar retrospective, fee-for-service method of reimbursement, you catch a feel for this revolution.) And DRGs are just the tip of the iceberg. Admissions, lengths of stay, and inpatient revenues are shrinking fast. It is estimated that the hospital's share of the health care market will decrease from 42 percent to 38 percent in the 1990s. Outpatient revenues are expected to double—from 13 percent to 25 percent. Our hospital marketing people tell me that half the hospitals in the United States lost money last year, leading to many closures (21 hospitals have closed in my home state of Illinois). All of this will lead hospitals to play vital but changed roles in the future.

Human suffering is not expected to decline. But where such people are treated, by whom, for how long, and at what cost will change dramatically. This varies from hospital to hospital, but where I work Medicare or Medicaid accounts for about 40 percent of our revenues; Blue Cross, 12 percent; commercial carriers, 36 percent; self-paying patients and others, 9 percent and managed care (via HMO/PPO), 4 percent. It is expected that in the 1990s managed care will increase to 25 percent of our reimbursements. Currently, managed care payers reimburse us for only 82 percent of the charges of our services. Because the market is so competitive, such managed care payers can drive a hard bargain. As their numbers and influence grow, they will drive even harder bargains. The possibilities for hospitals to shift costs—as they have done in the past—will be more limited. If, or when, Medicare or Medicaid and managed care reimbursers come to represent 65–75 percent of a hospital's revenues, cost shifting will be impossible.

Declining reimbursements will intensify the internal competition for those reduced budgetary dollars. Chaplaincy is not being singled out in cost reductions but is at a sharp disadvantage in not being a direct revenue producer or having its services mandated by hospital accreditation bodies or state licensing agencies. As Peggy Way has put it, "Chaplains always function in someone else's institutions."[3] Consequently, we are always a little out of place in terms of power, ownership, authority, and location. "We function by someone else's sufferance, under someone else's authority, enabled by someone else's resources."[4]

If your hospital and you as a chaplain have not been affected by these socioeconomic changes, then you really are in heaven. And you should know it.

Where Does This Leave the Chaplain?

Like hospitals, it leaves us as chaplains with a changed, but vital role. Being part of the health care establishment that is undergoing marked changes, we chaplains cannot expect to be, and will not be, immune to those changes. However, chaplaincy will survive this revolution. We must, we have too much at stake; we have worked too hard and are too valuable a resource not to survive. Our roles may need to be redefined, our context will diversify, our numbers may shrink—but we will persevere. We chaplains will not become an endangered species; but we will need to adapt to these changes:

Sicker Patients and Shorter Hospital Stays (5.5 days on average). Hospital admissions will drop from 138 per 1,000 to 129 per 1,000 in the early 1990s. Declines will come, in part, because more patients can expect to pay first-dollar coverage and larger deductibles to discourage overutilization.

Discharge planning will begin with the initial hospital visit. Short-term ministries will need to be implemented. To bridge the parenthesis of hospitalization (soon to average less than a week), tie-ins with local parishes, families, community agencies, and discharge planning personnel will be mandatory.

Older Patients. Every day 5,000 people in the U.S. turn 65. In our country there are more people over 65 than under 20. By 1995 those over 65 will comprise 13 percent of the population; by 2030 it will be 21 percent—about 66 million. By that year the ratio between children under 18 and those over 65 will be 1 to 1. Also by 2030, the ratio of active workers to retired citizens will slip from 6 to 1 (where it is today) to 3 to 1. We will soon be the first society in history to have two generations of the same family in retirement and on Social Security and Medicare. These elderly will provide about two-thirds of hospitals' revenues. Currently we allocate 30 percent of our health care resources for those in the last years of their lives. A majority of these people are elderly. A further complication has been government underpayment for Medicare patients. Yet these underpayments have not been accompanied by cutbacks in demand. Just the opposite. In its first year (1965), Medicare cost $4.7 billion, less than 3 percent of the federal budget to cover 19 million people.[5] Today it consumes 7 percent of our federal budget to cover 30 million people.

Enormous challenges confront us through this growing segment of our population. DRGs are forcing many of the patients to go home sooner than expected, sooner than they and their families are prepared for discharge.

Indigent, Underinsured Patients. It is estimated that 33–37 million Americans are without health coverage in the United States, many of them children. If you add to this those who are considered underinsured, it raises the figure to about one in four Americans. These are people who fall through the gaps. Uninsured care is estimated to cost $6 billion annually—or 1–4 percent of a hospital's revenues, depending upon the hospital's location. Uncollected patient revenues are expected to swell to 5–10 percent in the 1990s. The non- and underinsured tend not to seek medical care until they have to, which makes their care even more extensive when they seek it.

In any market-driven system, logic would say to avoid such nonpaying customers, yet most of us are from church hospitals, whose mission ought to embrace such people. But someone has to pay. Like all competitive services, it appears inevitable that we will be compelled to devise a multitiered delivery system. The payer will simply not stand for open access to the system by the nonpayer.

It is reluctantly acknowledged that in the next decade the uninsured, without ability to pay, will experience the greatest decline in quantity and quality of health services. And, unlike the elderly, the poor have little political clout.

Overworked, Burned-Out Staffs. As staffs grow smaller and the need for productivity increases, hospital personnel will be required to do more with less. It will be extremely important for hospitals to recruit, train, and retain competent and dedicated people. Stress and burnout will be endemic.

Stress occurs when our capacities to adapt are consistently overtaxed; burnout results when our caring capacities are overstretched, with seemingly little return experienced on our emotional investment. Given this high-pressure, demanding environment, chaplains may be asked to spend as much time with staffs as with patients, helping them to cope more effectively with stress and burnout.

For all our talk about cost containment, efficiency, and productivity, it will be vital that hospitals keep the personal dimension of health care in perspective. It is a high-tech and high-touch enterprise. This will be vital for two important reasons: (1) healing, in the fuller sense of the word, derives more from personal than technical care, and (2) most patients, being unable to evaluate technical competency, will judge the hospital's efforts by whether or not they felt personally regarded.

Mounting Demands to Monitor Quality and Measure Outcomes of Our Pastoral Services. The "in" word these days is outcome, not services. Outcome will be measured by very tangible means. Length of stay, recidivism, return to work, and cost. The question will be, Is this service a legitimate health care expense, or does it merely contribute to quality of life? It is expected that third-party payers will reward health care in the most narrow sense: accurate diagnosis and documented treatment plans, that which is medically prescribed and closely reviewed. Any services that do not fit those narrow categories will face challenge. As George Caldwell, the former president and chief executive officer of, and now a consultant for, the Lutheran General Health Care System, Park Ridge, Illinois, laments, "Hospitals are in danger of becoming body shops."

This will raise some very basic and serious questions for and about pastoral care, having to do with the intent and nature of our services, our goals, our credentials, and our capacity to document outcome.

What kinds of outcome indicators can we turn to in pastoral care? Do we learn the new language, define monitoring tools, and seek to measure outcome and thereby run the risk of reducing our ministry—a ministry that relies on interpersonal relationships, process, and internal growth—to pragmatic, functional, measurable results? Can we? Should we? Can we afford not to?

Do chaplains stand up to the pressures by insisting that spiritual faith has its own rewards, whether or not it contributes toward a favorable medical outcome, but in so doing insulate our services from everyone's scrutiny and possibly jeopardize our budgets?

It is a difficult dilemma, but an unavoidable one.

Marketplace Ethics. It appears that tomorrow's ethical clashes will take place in boardrooms and administrative offices, and only indirectly at bedsides. The questions will have to do with resource distribution, medical rationing, balancing quality with affordability. The key players will be administrators, comptrollers, and hospital boards as well as legislatures. These people will need to make decisions without the benefit of long-standing, historic, professional codes of ethics (such as the Hippocratic oath, Florence Nightingale pledge, ordination covenants) that have evolved over centuries and provided value systems for doctors, nurses, and chaplains. Administrators and financiers will need to forge their codes of ethics on the run.

Ethical tensions will sharpen between managers and clinicians over priorities and the distribution of health care resources and conflicts over the competing claims of individual patients versus institutional survival. Chaplains may, by tradition and function, find themselves walking between these clinical and nonclinical worlds, helping each to face and accept the moral legitimacy of both commitments.

In this process, we chaplains may find ourselves spending more time with our administrators, helping them and our hospitals to identify more clearly our institutional goals, identity, values, vision, role, and mission. For without such clarity, our hospitals can easily be captured by market imperatives alone. Chaplains need to symbolize and bring to that business ethic the imperatives of the gospel, which include compassion and concern for the outcast, the oppressed, and social justice.

In a sense, we must walk between the worlds of faith and finance. I am not suggesting that quality, efficiency, productivity, and profit are antithetical to the gospel, but that they must be held in juxtaposition to a hospital's mission. We will need to help our hospitals to be *bifocal,* looking not only at the bottom lines, but also at the top lines of value and vision, and *bilingual,* familiar not with the language of markets but also with the languages of mercy, faith, and caring.

Like the stewards in Jesus' parable of the talents (Matt. 25:14-30), chaplains may need to challenge their employer hospitals to be both diligent (that is, fiscally prudent) and faithful (to their commitment to serve suffering people of all classes, colors, and needs).

Efficiency and mission are mutually dependent. If our employer hospitals fail financially, their loftiest missions will be of little avail. But if technical and financial success are the only barometers, their mission will be superfluous. "For what does it profit any individual or institution to gain the whole world and to lose its soul?"

What is and will be needed is the chaplain's prophetic voice in helping our hospitals confront the inevitable yet intrinsic conflicts between mission and profit, between human services and the bottom line.

Walter Brueggemann speaks of the prophetic role as both criticizing and energizing.[6] We need to be courageous (for no prophet ever brings an unconflicted, harmonious message) and visionary (for no prophet ever gets beset by those conflicts). We need to help find answers, not just point out problems.

Transcending Hospital Borders and Ministering to Suffering People in a Variety of Environments in a Variety of Ways. As hospitals must move beyond the narrow inpatient parameters of care, so must chaplains. This is because in the past, we and they have been predominantly inpatient focused. This made sense for several reasons:

1. It was convenient—the patient did the traveling.

2. It was consistent with the hospital's focus and reimbursement system, since inpatients were the source of our hospitals' revenues and were thereby most entitled to our services.

3. It saved time. It was possible to see more people over shorter periods when they were concentrated in one building.

4. Inpatients were a captive audience, and therefore easier to reach. In addition to receiving technologic and medical services, they were "hotel guests," in need of food, clean rooms, entertainment, and companionship. In many instances the technical

care they received occupied only a sliver of their total time spent in the hospital.

Yet we always knew that significant—if not the most significant—healing took place after hospitalization, back in the home and community. We knew that our ministry was at best very limited and tangential. We often envied the parish clergy and family physicians who had access to these people prior to, and following, that narrow parenthesis of hospitalization.

Many broken people who used to be in our hospitals will not be there tomorrow. They will be in outpatient facilities, hospices, birthing centers, ambulatory surgical centers, emergency rooms, at home.

It is interesting how the pendulum is swinging again. At the turn of the 20th century, hospitals were not the best place for sick people. They were havens for infection. People were better off at home, amidst the tender, loving care of family. Hospitals tended to house the poor or those who lacked such family support. For vastly different reasons, more medical care will return to the home and the family. It is not that hospitals are unsafe today; they are too expensive, at least by economic priorities we have set as a nation.

Medically, we are creatively finding new ways to do old things in different settings.

The Outpatient Scene

A revolutionary expansion of outpatient services is upon us. Again, we may be too close to it to fully appreciate its scope and implications. Inpatient acute care will become just one segment of a diverse health care enterprise, and not necessarily its hub. We are doing more complicated procedures on sicker patients in outpatient settings. Volume and revenues are increasing, accounting for as much as 20–25 percent of a hospital's income. We are quickly coming to realize that inpatient services need not be the exclusive mode of health care or pastoral care. Within 10 years, it is estimated that 70 percent of health care services will be provided outside the hospital.

Ambulatory surgery is leading the way in many hospitals. (At my hospital, outpatient surgery accounts for about 40 percent of all surgical procedures.) In outpatient surgery we bind lesions, remove moles and cataracts, do tonsillectomies, breast biopsies, arthroscopies, laryngoscopies, esophagostomies, hemorrhoidectomies, D & Cs, some hernia surgery, plastic surgery, and infertility procedures, as well as change pacemakers. Surgeons tell me outpatient hysterectomies, appendectomies, and cholecystectomies are just around the corner.

The clinical load of Lutheran General's gastrointestinal (GI) lab has more than doubled in the past five years. Almost half of its work is now treatment: laser therapy for cancer of the esophagus, radiation of bronchial tumors, and removal of polyps. And they attempt to diagnose abdominal pains of unknown origin, emergency bleeding, and other intestinal blockages with sigmoidoscopies, gastroscopies, and endoscopies.

At our hospital, we have radiation therapy and nuclear medicine; an outpatient cancer care unit; cardiac lab and heart stations that give stress tests, electrocardiograms, and magnetic resonance imaging; a lithotripter (to crush kidney stones); laproscopic laser techniques that enable surgeons to visualize and remove a gall bladder or an appendix without opening the abdomen; a psychiatric outpatient clinic; a day hospital; a day center for older adults; respiratory care for chronic respiratory and emphysema patients; a home care or hospice program; physical, occupational, and speech therapy; an active emergency room with a trauma center (from which only about 27 percent are admitted as inpatients); plus a variety of outpatient services, including blood transfusions, intravenous therapy, catheter insertion, EEGs, sleep laboratories, and diabetic counseling. I suspect most hospitals in this nation could compile a similar array of outpatient services. The list keeps growing. This movement, in the view of Gerald McManis, a Washington-based health care consultant, is more than a matter of shifting traditional services and costs from an inpatient to an outpatient setting. There will be new businesses and services requiring creative approaches and demanding different managerial skills.[7]

Such growth has produced problems, the major one being the slowness of all of us (pastoral care personnel included) to respond. Most hospitals do not see themselves as outpatient facilities. Their reputations were built on inpatient critical care. In addition, hospitals have been forced to adapt institutions built for inpatients for use by outpatients. This has resulted in many problems that are too familiar to most hospital-based outpatient services, namely:

- A lack of space and privacy to be prepped for procedures, await procedures, consult with one's physicians, to secure valuables like purses, billfolds, and watches (last year our hospital paid out $16,000 on lost personal property claims);
- confusion about access, slow registration, and inadequate, inconvenient parking;
- facilities scattered throughout the hospital often requiring walks down long corridors;
- unfriendly billing systems that sometimes require up-front payments and reimbursement systems that are not always clear about what outpatient services are covered;
- a feeling of being hustled out of the hospital before the patient and family feel discharge is warranted.

While enjoying the mobility and the freedom to come and go the same day, outpatients also feel they are left more on their own with regard to payments, verifying insurance coverage, and managing their own care.

Although many diagnostic and treatment procedures are now quicker and seemingly done with less fuss and bother, the anxieties and uncertainties of outcome, the threats, and pains are the same for outpatients as inpatients. In addition, patients in outpatient facilities are sicker than they were years ago. There seems little question that technical quality is not being compromised in outpatient services, but there is serious question as to whether the fuller support systems—including pastoral care—are as available to outpatients. Hospitals and third-party reimbursers know we can provide lower-cost treatment to outpatients, but are these services always humane and sensitive?

The one consolation is the more obvious presence of the family. For many outpatient procedures (such as ambulatory surgery), a friend or family member must accompany the patient to provide support and transportation. So patients come to rely more upon their real, rather than a contrived, support system.

Outpatients provide some problems for pastoral caregivers, particularly in the area of access. They are much harder to connect with. Unlike inpatients, most of their time spent in the outpatient facility will be occupied by technological procedures—whether diagnostic or therapeutic. There is little slack time in the process, except when they are waiting in line or sitting in a lobby. It is difficult to isolate the patient from a congested environment.

In addition, the mind-set of the outpatient is to get the procedure done and get out of the building. It is not a situation conducive to patients' reflecting upon their feelings, their life, or crisis. There is little time for such things and little opportunity to develop any significant bonding between patient and chaplain under such time and space pressures. Such relationships have an uncertain beginning and little formal closure.

Outpatient ministry also calls for different skills: a bolder, more aggressive approach, requiring a gregarious person who meets people easily and puts them at ease. It is a ministry that demands spontaneity and flexibility, since it is difficult to structure such encounters.

Yet these are contextual issues that do not, and should not, diminish the pastoral role or the theological validation for ministry in outpatient settings where suffering people are found.

Just as many of us wondered if we could make the adjustment from parish to hospital ministry, where we had only an average seven- to nine-day hospitalization parenthesis, now we face a ministry that is encapsulated not in days or hours, but in minutes.

The Challenge of Outpatient
Ministry for Pastoral Care

To know that emotional-spiritual needs are as present in outpatients as inpatients and to confront the logistical difficulties of engaging those needs are both the frustration and challenge for pastoral care today. It is a frustration and a challenge we can ill afford to ignore if we are to remain relevant to our hospitals. And while professional survival ought not to be our driving force, we in chaplaincy recognize the imperative to adapt to a radically new medical environment.

I propose we employ the following six strategies to meet the challenge more adequately.

1. *Learn more about outpatients—who they are and what they need.* We need to spend time talking to our outpatient staffs and

learning of their needs, as well as their perceptions of outpatients' needs. We should arrange to spend time in various outpatient settings, visit with patients and families, encourage and help our administrations to develop and send out patient-satisfaction questionnaires to help identify the strengths and weaknesses of our institutions' outpatient service delivery, and work with outpatient staffs in pulling together focus groups of those who recently received outpatient services. Let the "experts"—the outpatients themselves—tell you what it is all about.

2. *Play a prophetic role in trying to represent the concerns of outpatients and outpatient staffs to the administration.* In most hospitals much remains to be done to reshape a focus upon outpatients. This gets back to some problems identified earlier—ease of access, reducing red tape, consolidating facilities, simplifying the billing system, expanding convenient parking, and providing more space and privacy.

Supporting such environmental changes in any way the chaplain can is truly a form of pastoral care—on behalf of patients, families, and outpatient staffs.

3. *Take initiatives that are practical and possible.* Given the time pressures already cited, there seems no way that a chaplain can expect to take geographic initiatives with outpatients comparable to those with inpatients. The outpatient context is too prohibitive. A better use of time would be to work with outpatient staffs—identify your availability and services, suggest situations and ways you might be of service to their outpatients.

Develop an attractive brochure that defines you and your services and make it available to outpatients and families.

Periodically but regularly show up in those outpatient areas where you think your ministry has the greatest chance of being utilized. In pastoral care we have much history to support the notion that visibility leads to utilization.

Focus your energies upon patients who will be in some form of sustained outpatient care (such as patients with AIDS, cancer, heart disease, renal dialysis, parents of newborns with congenital anomalies, and psychiatric patients).

Focus your energies upon families. Though the patient may be totally consumed in receiving technical services, families are not. They have the time, they have needs, and they are accessible.

In other words, chaplains have limited amounts of time for geographic initiatives in outpatient areas. We will need to use such time prudently and efficiently. We cannot be everywhere. We will need to assess which outpatient areas offer the best possibilities for ministry.

4. *Expand outpatient services from existing inpatient services.* This has occurred quite spontaneously in Lutheran General. We make preoperative visits to all patients who go to surgery (usually the evening before surgery), so it was a natural extension to assign a chaplain to visit patients who come in the day of surgery. It means an early morning start for that chaplain.

We have a chaplain on cancer care. That ministry flowed naturally into our newly established Cancer Outreach Program (where she now spends 40 percent of her time) and to our Hospice/Home Care Program (which consumes about 10 percent of her time).

We are called for all hospital deaths. So it seemed logical to develop outpatient grief groups for such families (we now have six groups) and to conduct bimonthly memorial services.

We have a director of parish relations whose presence led to a parish nurse program that now includes 13 nurses working as ministers of health in 17 local parishes. The participating parishes and our hospital share the costs.

Isolated post-hospital counseling sessions between discharged patients and our pastoral care staff evolved quite naturally into a pastoral counseling center that currently has a staff of 16 full-time, AAPC (American Association of Pastoral Counselors)—certified counselors and 19 students, who in 1989 provided 19,500 clinical hours of outpatient visits. Most referrals have come from community parishes.

Likewise, our chaplain on the coronary units coleads a Mended Hearts Group, our psychiatric chaplain spends time in our day hospital, and our chaplain on the rehabilitation unit follows some patients who return for physical or occupational therapy.

Many ministries initiated on inpatient units have evolved slowly into outpatient services. We do not give such services the time and staff they deserve, but they are a start.

5. *Form liaisons with parish clergy.* As more care is shifted out of the hospital into the home, from the professional caregiver to

the family, opportunities abound for us to work more closely with the community, particularly parish pastors. Whether it be through more deliberate referrals, providing parish clergy easier entries to our outpatient service areas, or helping them to mobilize and train lay volunteers to assist families in their increased caring functions, much needs to be done. More than in recent memory, the parish clergy will be thrust more dynamically into the healing ministry of parishioners who will find themselves with less extensive support from physicians, nurses, and hospitals.

6. *Form liaisons with larger primary care medical practices.* Doctors' offices are changing in the midst of all these other changes. Many are integrating their medical services to include lab work, X rays, minor surgeries, casting and splinting, physical therapy—so why not pastoral care? There is bonding between those patients and that physician group practice, as there probably is between those physicians and the hospital.

This panel of physicians would, no doubt, be part of an HMO. A liaison between chaplains and such a group could certainly tighten the physician bond with the hospital and enable that physician group to broaden its services in a unique way.

Costs could be absorbed by the practice itself, with some direct billing to patients, or could be shared with the hospital. Closer ties between physicians and hospitals—and less competition—will need to occur in the changing medical world of the future. Such ties can be reciprocally rewarding for both hospital and physician.

In thinking of outpatient ministry, it will be necessary for us to make some ventures into primary care sites outside the hospital. Throughout most of our history, we chaplains have worked closely with physicians but our location, administrative ties, and salaries have been in, with, and from hospitals. Forming liaisons with primary care physician groups may be the creative thrust of the future.

Conclusion

Health care is in crisis. Chaplaincy is in crisis. Changes and threats abound. The challenges and opportunities are compelling. Though much of the motivation for outpatient services came through technological and market imperatives, such approaches may turn out to be in the patient's best interest. Surely they reduce some of the institutional dependency that inpatient services foster.

But what may be best for the patient complicates our ministry and has forced us into the new, less familiar world of the outpatient. Maybe in all of these disruptions we can feel a deeper kinship with patients, who are also in crisis.

• Like patients, we chaplains yearn for those good ol' pre-crisis days, when our work environment was more predictable.
• Like patients, we face boundaries and limits.
• Like patients, we face ominous dangers to old patterns and lively opportunities for new growth and vitality.
• Like the patients to whom we minister, we chaplains will need new visions and the will and courage to pursue them.

Notes

1. Joseph Califano, Jr., *America's Health Care Revolution: Who Lives, Who Dies, Who Pays?* (New York: Random House, 1986), 30.

2. Daniel Callahan, *What Kind of Life: The Limits of Medical Progress* (New York: Simon & Schuster, 1990), 71.

3. Peggy Way, unpublished remarks given at the annual convention of the American Association of Clinical Pastoral Education, Philadelphia, Penn., 1987.

4. Ibid.

5. Califano, *America's Health Care Revolution*, 140.

6. Walter Brueggemann, *The Prophetic Imagination* (Philadelphia: Fortress Press, 1978), 13.

7. Gerald McManis, "Viewpoint: Challenges of New Decade Demand Break with Tradition," in *Modern Health Care*, 8 Jan. 1990, 60.

Chapter 3

THE CHAPLAIN'S
OUTPATIENT MINISTRY

I. Introduction
By Ronald H. Sunderland

Directors of hospital pastoral care departments tend to communicate the expectation to their staffs that within reasonable limits, all patients are to receive the ministries of the department. That expectation is increasingly compromised by budgetary restraints limiting the number of chaplains in institutions, by factors that restrict hospitalization to more acute medical needs, and by the growing numbers of people who are being treated in outpatient clinics. Chaplains appointed to visit in clinics are likely to be confronted with large numbers of outpatients, all listening for their names to be called by the clinic staff, and each surrounded by walls of anxiety, feeling the need for privacy, and ambivalent about permitting intrusion into that privacy.

The Daunting Nature of the Task

The essays that follow report the experiences of four staff chaplains at the University of Texas M. D. Anderson Cancer Center in Houston, where more and more procedures are done in outpatient clinics. The staff chaplains initiated a study program to ascertain how best to offer pastoral care in this burgeoning setting. The essays attempt to identify pastoral "problems" that inhibit ministry, and do not so much offer resolutions as invite the reader to struggle with the authors in seeking those resolutions.

One of the first discoveries we made was the daunting volume of patients in most of the clinics, the difficulty (and often the impossibility) of securing any sense of privacy for pastoral conversations, the preoccupation of patients with hearing and responding to calls for them to present at the clinic desk, and their not surprising wish or need to leave the clinic at the first available opportunity and return to the refuges of their homes.

The second discovery was that outpatient ministry differs from inpatient pastoral care in many ways, and there were times—and days—when each of us preferred the latter assignments. We concluded that visits to inpatients are "easier" than those to outpatients! It is probably accurate to report that in our various ways, we felt somewhat guilty about our ambivalence. But we found we were not alone in these feelings; clinical pastoral education (CPE) students in the hospital training program, assigned to both inpatient and outpatient units, seemed to spend over 90 percent of their time at patients' bedsides, although the numbers of patients in the clinics far outweigh numbers of inpatients.

To Be or Not to Be . . . an Outpatient Chaplain

It was the realization of our ambivalence toward outpatient assignments that forced us to examine the entire kaleidoscope of outpatient ministry. Nathan Huang recounted his first experience as a lay assistant in a mission congregation in California 25 years earlier, remembering that although some people were friendly and receptive, others were rude and mean. The fear that he felt then still wells up in him whenever he enters a clinic.

With reality staring us in the face, we knew as chaplains we had no choice: it is not just that clinics are here to stay—they are rapidly expanding. The question was not "Is there a place for us as outpatient chaplains?" but "How do we minister in these clinics?" Virgil Fry put it succinctly: We are not talking about a few doctors' offices and laboratories and a handful of adjoining hospital rooms. We are talking major medical centers; alteration of traditional inpatient care to outpatient care; and high-tech diagnostic capabilities that stagger the mind and strain the budget. CAT scans, laser surgeries, and physical therapy are no longer confined to hospitals—the clinic has its own. In many hospitals, the clinic has become the hub of medical, surgical, and psychiatric care.

The Chaplain as Listener

Huang has found that the most effective way of beginning his day is to make his presence known to the desk staff, greet the first patient or family member nearest the counter. He introduces himself and asks if there is anything he can do while they are waiting for their appointment. Most people are pleased to learn chaplains are assigned to the clinics.

Many pastoral conversations are short, often interrupted, and with little or no opportunity for follow-up care. The chaplain must become accustomed to conversing with the patient while both are listening for the desk clerks' announcements. Conversations are often half finished, "unsatisfactory," or what Dietrich Bonhoeffer called "pen-ultimate" ministries.

The "Waiting" Room

A stanza from Henry Wadsworth Longfellow's poem "Resignation" identifies one of the most grievous aspects of outpatient care:

> Let us, then, be up and doing,
>   With a heart for any fate;
> Still achieving, still pursuing,
>   Learn to labor and to wait.

The time patients spend "waiting" for medical care remains one of the burdens not only for the patients caught up in the clinic process, but for any sensitive staff member. Yet clinic staff may become so used to this additional stress upon patients that it is too easily overlooked as the inevitable and inescapable cost of being seen as an outpatient. It is when one sits where patients sit that the frustration is shared. Fry tells about sitting for an hour in a clinic station waiting to see a family who had requested pastoral care. As time went by, his frustration rose. Soon he became aware of his hostility, frustration, despair, the unfairness of the situation, and just good old-fashioned anger. But during the hour he waited, he refocused his perspective: there is treachery in being a patient or family member with very little control over scheduling, procedures, or the medical condition responsible for bringing the patient to the clinic in the first place.

Inpatients are often accompanied by family members, and the chaplain's ministry frequently includes them. In some instances, the only contact a chaplain may have is with a family member, but frequently there are opportunities for extended conversations with the patient alone. Outpatients almost invariably are accompanied by family members or friends who drove them to the hospital clinic, dropped them at the front door, parked the car, located them at one of their clinic stops, brought coffee from the cafeteria, and then sit, also waiting, until the ordeal is over. Family members may assist in making the next appointment, and help patients understand what the doctor said, perhaps correcting the patients' perceptions. Family members often appreciate a chaplain's willingness to listen as they weigh options and ponder aloud the "what ifs."

Ministry in the Ambulatory Surgery Clinic

Little is to be gained by comparing the services of one clinic with those of another. Each clinic population faces its own level of stress, and the observer is hardly in a position to gauge which patient or group of patients face the greater level of threat. Yet in a sense there is something unique about the same-day surgery setting, at least in a major cancer center, where many procedures accompanied by high levels of stress are performed. Geri Opsahl has ministered to patients who are veterans of their fight against cancer as well as others who are novices.

Opsahl proposes two models for pastoral ministry in this setting. The "external" model focuses on the supportive, more visible role of the chaplain. It calls on the chaplain to *do* things for patients and families and so is attractive; one often feels better when *doing* something. The four functions follow:

1. *Providing information.* Research has demonstrated that patients experience a greater degree of control when they are well informed about hospital procedures. In turn, the sense of degree of control complements not only intrapsychic health but also physical health.

2. *Offering reassurance.* For those facing surgery, waiting seems unbearable. The chaplain's presence can serve to calm them, to release tension, and to hold up hope.

3. *Providing communication.* As the day progresses, the chaplain serves as liaison between patients in recovery and families in the waiting area and, on occasion, between medical staff and families.

4. *Offering support.* The chaplain supports patients in recovery both by listening to them and enabling them to communicate with their waiting families. Perhaps the most pain-filled moments are those in which the chaplain accompanies a surgeon who provides a report to a waiting family or to the patient. People who receive good news do so in the context of their awareness that many patients will not be so fortunate, and may experience feelings of guilt because of their joy, or because they feel unworthy of receiving it. Patients and families receiving an unfavorable report are reassured that the chaplain will walk with them through the dark times they are facing.

Opsahl's second model, the "internal" model, refers to the motivation of the chaplain's ministry. There are four components:

1. *Sensitivity.* People in the waiting area are extremely vulnerable; their sense of mastery has evaporated, and their personhood is open and unguarded. Chaplains need to approach them with tender, loving care.

2. *Intentionality.* The purposefulness of the chaplain both strengthens the offering of pastoral care and alerts giver and receiver that the chaplain is not merely a passive presence, but makes a positive contribution.

3. *Visibility.* Henry Nouwen has an interesting thesis about being "present." The ministry of presence, Nouwen claims, needs to be balanced by the "ministry of absence. This is because it

belongs to the essence of a creative ministry constantly to convert the pain of the Lord's absence into a deeper understanding of his presence. *But absence can only be converted if it is first of all experienced.*"[1] Readers familiar with Nouwen's concept will remember that he goes on to suggest that there is a ministry in which "our leaving creates space" for God's Spirit and in which, by our absence, God can become present in a new way. But he dramatizes his point by adding: "There is an enormous difference between an absence *after* a visit and an absence which is the result of *not coming at all* (our emphases). Without a coming, there can be no leaving, and without a presence absence is only emptiness and not the way to a greater intimacy with God through the Spirit."[2]

It is this ministry of "presence" and "absence" that the chaplain brings to the outpatient clinic. The chaplain's presence consists of two elements, intrinsic and extrinsic: The physical presence of the chaplain in the clinic witnesses to the concern of the sponsoring religious agency (judicatory, department of pastoral care) and the hospital's concern to provide such a ministry in response to the patients' and families' needs and concerns. The physical presence is accompanied by the chaplain's words of support and compassion.

The chaplain's presence also has a symbolic meaning. The mere presence of the religious community's representative is a reminder of the meanings and values espoused by that community, and reminds patients and families of their ties to their respective faith groups. The chaplain's presence is not coercive, but embodies an invitation to each person present to call on the resources of the religious community, or to inquire about them. It states that these resources are freely accessible to all present.

4. *Readiness.*   All of the elements of ministry previously identified imply that the chaplain must be alert to opportunities for ministry, aware of the nuances implicit (sometimes explicit) in patients' or family members' inquiries and messages, and able to interpret these messages so as to respond in the manner appropriate to the person's inner needs. Opsahl identifies this aspect of ministry as "serendipity," urging chaplains to be on the lookout for the presence of something valuable that was not sought or

expected, making the adventure of outpatient ministry the setting for "grace-filled moments."

In the closing chapter in this section, Sister Margaret Whooley reflects on her ministry. She wonders if she is willing, available, and vulnerable to take the risk, to evoke the potential of persons to be part of their own healing, and to connect their wounds to the wounds of all humanity and with the suffering servant of God. She recalled the way a dying 54-year-old man and his agitated wife gratefully received care and became more peaceful. A key to outpatient ministry is the presence of healing relationships on individual, family, and institutional levels.

II. Outpatient Family Needs
By Virgil Fry

The Clinic. The word itself sounds institutional and sterile. It smacks of an intrusion into normal daily life. So lacking in warmth or any touch except medical. So busy, so impersonal, so, well, clinical.

We are not talking about a few doctors' offices and laboratories and a handful of adjoining hospital rooms. We are talking about major medical centers. We are talking about alteration of traditional inpatient care to outpatient care. We are talking about high-tech diagnostic capabilities that stagger the mind and strain the budget. CAT scans, laser surgeries, and physical therapy are no longer confined to hospitals—the clinic has come into its own.

For many major and midsized hospitals, the clinic has become the hub of medical, surgical, and psychiatric care. Outpatient diagnosis and treatment is preferred by insurance companies, patients, and reluctantly, the medical community. The army's motto of "hurry up and wait" has become the unofficial creed of clinics. People resist being a number on a medical assembly line of unpredictable news.

Significant others, the catchphrase of institutions, are also part of the clinic scene. Family members and supportive friends walk clinic halls and occupy seats in waiting rooms. They serve as encouragers and enablers. They provide a link of safety and concern in a threatening environment of strangers wearing white coats and stethoscopes. They have a vital function in the clinic.

Several months ago I sat for an hour in a clinic station waiting to minister to a patient and family who had contacted me. As I debated whether to wait for the physician to complete his treatment with the patient or to leave, I resolved to stay. After all, it should only be a few minutes, right? After 15 minutes, my frustration level increased. Again I considered my options. Again I chose to stay. After all, the clinic had already cost me 15 valuable minutes!

Forty-five minutes later, I was still waiting. Being aware of my inner feelings during experiences was part of my chaplaincy training. In this instance, my C.P.E. training was not in vain. I was in touch with my hostility, frustration, despair, sense of unfairness, and good old-fashioned anger. That hour I refocused my perspective. It is treacherous to be a patient or family member with very little control over scheduling, procedures, or the medical condition that was responsible for bringing the person here in the first place. My thoughts returned to an earlier time when I was a family member in a similar "hurry up and wait" environment. My frustration from those past experiences carried over to this clinic where I was a chaplain, not a family member.

During that hour, I saw three doctors enter the nurses' station and request to see one particular patient. A nurse entered the waiting room, asked the family where the patient was, and suggested the family go retrieve him from the cafeteria. The appointment was not for another 30 minutes, but the medical team was present and wanted to see a body. The family fulfilled the request.

Another man, pushing a woman in a wheelchair to the clerk's desk, said loudly: "My wife's been here since 1:00 P.M." I looked at my watch—it was now 4:00 P.M. This woman had waited three hours in a wheelchair, and yet I was upset at 15 minutes in a cushioned chair I could easily have abandoned.

I scanned the waiting room full of people. Some sat and stared. Some slept. Some read magazines. Some showed obvious discomfort. Some conversed. Some made future appointments. Some were told to go back and "get your chart."

The clinic. The crossroads of scientific objective data and human beings. It is here that shocking, life-changing words are pronounced. Words like:

"This will sting a little," or

"I'm referring you to a specialist," or

"Is any of your family with you?" or

"It doesn't look good," or

"You need to be admitted into the hospital," or

"It's cancer," "It's your heart," "It's MS," "It's benign," or

"Surgery, chemo, and radiation are your only options," or

"You've got a 50–50 chance," or

"Do you have any questions?"

Family members are left—or expected—to pick up the pieces. Family members help set the next appointment. Family members walk the patient to the car. Family members help decipher what was actually said versus what the patient and family wanted to hear. Family members help weigh options and ponder aloud the "what ifs."

Sometimes family members are asked by the medical team to pressure a patient into a certain treatment. Recently, a friend in the clinic was explaining to me her decision to pursue no further treatment. After six years, four recurrences, and no blood counts, she was determined to go home. She wished to live life to its fullest, then seek hospice care. Her doctor's advice when informed of her refusal of further chemotherapy was, "Go call your husband, and let him talk you into taking it."

Often family members silently cope with anger, guilt, denial, and disbelief. God is pleaded with and cursed in the same breath. Family roles are played out in exaggerated form. Hoping to lessen painful reality, the family may erect a protective wall around the patient. Doctors, nurses, lab techs, and chaplains are instructed what to say and what to avoid saying. Sometimes the family finds the news too overwhelming and leaves the patient alone. Sometimes family members ask unanswerable questions such as "why?" and "how long?"

What does the pastoral caregiver have to offer in such an environment? The answer is as diverse as the individuals to whom we are privileged to minister. Open arms and open hearts are the biblical model we invoke.

We can care enough to be present for the good news as well as the bad. We can provide a sense of openness that allows expression of feelings. We can avoid pat answers and glib advice. We can take a family member out for coffee, and more often than not, for a cry, a fist-banging, or a prayer. We can offer communication that listens to unrealistic hopes or despair. We can share pastoral concerns with the local church if appropriate. We can be flexible enough with our time to sense when it is best to stay longer than we intended.

In short, we can care. Our ministry is in being touched by another's struggle and responding with a touch of community. It is the same ministry that is needed in the hospital room, the prison, or the shelter for the homeless and abused. It is loving because we have been loved. It is affirming that faith, hope, and love will abide in spite of the storm. It is treating a human being in the same significant way I need to be treated when the doctor tells me or my family, "There's nothing more we can do."

III. Clinic Station 80
By Nathan Huang

When I first came to this clinic station, I was frightened by the large number of patients and family members in the waiting area. I did not know where to start or how to approach them.

I recalled my first experience of working for a mission congregation as a lay assistant in California 25 years ago. My daily duty was to canvas the neighborhood, knocking on doors. Some people were friendly and receptive, others were not. In fact, some were rude and mean. One afternoon when I approached a house on a corner, before I said anything, one of the men sitting in the driveway drinking beer shouted at me "What do you want?" I was so unnerved that I turned and left immediately. The same sort of fear wells up in me whenever I enter a clinic.

To gather my strength and courage every morning when I enter the clinic I go to the windows first and meditate for a while. Next I go to the receptionist, chatting with her for a few minutes, and then I turn around to greet the first patient (or family member) nearest the reception counter. I usually begin by introducing myself and saying, "I just want to stop by to say hello and see if there is anything I can do to help while you are waiting for your appointment." Most people are pleased to learn that we have the chaplaincy service in the clinic. Some immediately share their feelings with me; others may not but appreciate my presence.

During my three years of ministry here, only one or two patients have told me that they did not want to be bothered. The majority are open and eager to talk to me, telling me all about their diagnosis, their fear, and their apprehension.

One woman from Florida was scared and nervous when she first came to the clinic. She and her son were here alone—no friends, no relatives. When I stopped by to talk to her, she was glad that someone cared enough to do so. Then she started telling me with tears that when she was young, she was a beauty in her old country, Cuba. After she met and married an American businessman, she moved to the United States and enjoyed her life tremendously. Then her husband left her for another woman. They were divorced just a year earlier. After a few months of grief, she had begun to pick up the pieces. Then suddenly she was diagnosed with breast cancer. Within a couple of weeks, she came to M. D. Anderson Cancer Center for consultation and was scheduled to have a mastectomy. This was a great shock to her and the thing that she seemed to grieve most was that she was going to lose a part of her body and that she would, in her own mind, no longer be a whole woman or beautiful. A few days later, I accompanied her and her son until she was wheeled into the operating room. She gave me a hug and clung to me as if I was her only relative.

Of course, not all patients are that open and willing to talk. Some are reserved or too embarrassed to talk in front of the other people in the waiting room. If they do not want to talk, I do not push them. I just let them know that I am there to help if they ever need me.

Another example is a "Pentecostal" man who asked whether he could visit with me for a few minutes. He asked me whether I believed that God answered prayers. I said I did. Then he asked me why God did not answer his prayers when he prayed for his father. He told me that he was raised a Baptist but changed to

Pentecostal when his father was dying of cancer, hoping that the Pentecostal belief in faith healing would save his father. But his prayer was not answered. His father died and that hurt and disappointed him. Since then, he has been very bitter toward God. But now he himself is suffering from the same disease. "Is God punishing me?" he asked.

First I listened to his angry talk and then I assured him that God does not use cancer to punish him or anyone. I tried to help him deal with his anger by encouraging him to talk. I told him that it was OK to get angry at God. We were interrupted when he was called into the doctor's office, but a few minutes later he came out with a smile and said to me: "I know God answers prayers, but it may not be what I wanted." He left that day with a renewed faith, even though he had the same medical problem.

Every day I encounter many faith issues. I try to avoid any controversial discussions (like arguments with Jehovah Witnesses) and be with patients wherever their faith journey is. A man who confessed his past to me had been overwhelmed with guilt. He raised a lot of questions about sin and punishment. I tried to help him see the positive side of faith: God's love and forgiveness. Sometimes I encourage patients to talk about their guilt. It usually makes them feel better to vent their feelings.

One day I almost passed by a woman sitting quietly when it was my lunchtime. But I decided to stop to greet her. When I asked how she was, she started crying and telling me that she was so scared and anxious. Furthermore, she was still grieving over the death of her son who was murdered by a burglar. She cried and talked for about 45 minutes. It was a very moving experience to be with her. She needed a sympathetic ear to hear her out at that time.

Every day I try to reach out to everyone in the waiting area. If they do not want to talk, it is okay; if they do, I stay and listen. I remember one morning when a group of women from a local church came to sing Christmas carols. Most of those who were in the room really liked the singing, except a middle-aged woman. She was sitting there silently. After the women finished their singing, I asked her if she liked the caroling. She said no; it had triggered a lot of sad memories in her. She said it was a long story. When I said it must be difficult for her to talk about, she started crying. I stood there silently for a while. Then I asked her if I could just sit with her for a while. She said yes and motioned me to sit next to her. After a brief hesitation she started pouring out her heart to me. Within the last year she had suffered three major tragedies—her husband had left her, her mother had died of cancer, and her only daughter had announced after her mother's funeral that she was a lesbian and was going to live with another woman. On top of all of this, the woman is now suffering the same disease that her mother died of. She was scared and lonely. She did not have anyone to talk to. She kept saying that she was lonely. I was with her for nearly an hour. A few days later, she came to thank me for being with her in her time of need. She told our secretary that she had never told anyone about her tragedies before.

It has been a rewarding and challenging experience for me to minister to a houseful of strangers every day. I still feel apprehensive, but not frightened. Once I am there, I feel more relaxed, especially when I see some familiar faces. The longer I work there, the easier it is. I am quite proud of the fact that my ministry to the outpatients there has been recognized and appreciated not only by the patients and family members, but also by the doctors and other staff members.

IV. Same-Day Surgery Clinics
By Geri Opsahl

As the number of outpatient surgeries skyrockets daily in the United States, we are recognizing an immediate need for pastoral presence in same-day surgery clinics. I do not think every clinic needs a chaplain, but surgery has a particular intensity that demands our presence.

Each day at 6:30 A.M., chaplains arrive at Clinic 44 in M. D. Anderson Cancer Center to meet outpatients, inpatients, and their families. The fact that patients scheduled for less serious surgeries wait side by side with patients checking in for major surgeries offers its own dynamic. In a cancer hospital it is easy for outpatients to project that in a few weeks or months they could be

surgery inpatients. Such projection heightens anxiety. Here is
what I saw in the same-day surgery clinic:

Over here is a young woman, 23 years old with no
children, having a total hysterectomy.
There is a man having his voice box removed, speaking
his last words and they are to you.
A woman is here for exploratory surgery with all its
uncertainty.
A young man who came for a bone marrow transplant
was told that this is his last chance at life.
Across the room a young child waits for a leg amputation.
A woman facing major facial reconstruction looks sad.
An old man whose heart stopped during his last surgery
sits near her.

Some have driven all night to get here and arrive
exhausted.
Some have flown in from other states or other countries.
Some are alone.
Some have 15 family members with them.
Some speak English.
Some don't.
Some are veterans of the cancer process.
Some are novices.

Many are anxious and show it.
Many are anxious and can't show it, covering their
feelings with selective attention to medical details.
Many are truly not anxious, feeling either acceptance or
resignation.
But most feel overwhelmed. And underneath the sense of
being overwhelmed is usually some type of fear:
Fear of diagnosis.
Fear of going to sleep.
Fear of bad news.
Fear of losing control.
Fear of not being self-sufficient.
Fear of becoming someone they are not.
Fear that it's only the beginning.

One patient said, "It's like waiting for the ax to fall."

All around them are their families; family systems under a terrible strain. People are switching roles. The strong become weak; the weak become strong. Family foundations shake as they desperately try to restore personal and family equilibrium.

Enter the chaplain, with his or her own dynamic process in operation. Perhaps he or she has gotten a speeding ticket on the way to the hospital. Maybe the chaplain has been on call all night. In any case, both chaplain and patient have their own personal defenses securely in place. How then does an encounter take place? How does a meeting happen when the chaplain who desires to be an intimate spiritual caregiver is a virtual stranger? We now confront one of the first issues in pastoral care in clinics—intrusion. I struggle with it daily. Personal privacy is important to me, and I know that it is to many others. Of course, this issue is individual. It seems that the only way to confront it is to believe the risk is worth taking. It takes courage to move away from your own "safe place" to provide a "safe place" for others. My personal style is not to plunge in but to ease into another's life and to do so with continuing permission.

I suggest two models for clinic ministry, the external and the internal. In group dynamics they would be called content and process.

In the external model (fig. 1), people observe me as chaplain as I go about my work. I function observably in four ways:

First, I provide *information* about scheduling, procedures, and other caregivers. This often is a way to gain people's trust while allowing them to retain some feeling of control. It allows them to raise questions or clarify points made by a caregiver but not really understood.

Second, I offer *reassurance*. People are barely holding on to get through the day and through the surgery. The waiting seems unbearable. The presence of a chaplain can serve to calm them, to steady them, to release tension through pastoral conversation, and to hold up hope.

Third, as the day progresses, I begin to act as a *liaison* between families and patients in recovery rooms or between medical personnel and families. As the chaplain, I am seen as an integral member of the team.

The fourth function is *support*. By its nature, surgery engenders high stress levels. When bad news is given, the chaplain often is present in the consultation room. People need support even when good news is given because they may feel guilty for experiencing joy or think they are unworthy of receiving it.

In the second model (fig. 2), no one observes our actions as chaplains. This is the model that motivates our ministry.

Sensitivity is an important component because people in the waiting area are extremely vulnerable. Their sense of mastery is gone, their personhood unguarded. Patients have said to me: "I used to feel invincible, but I don't anymore." We have a great responsibility to "tread lightly" as we enter another's life. I have experienced in my own life what it feels like to be trodden upon, so I jealously guard others' fragile points.

Second, we need to enter with *intention*. We are not strictly a passive presence. Intentionality does not mean evangelizing but having an internal mind-set centered on the question "Where is God in all this?"

Third, *visibility* is essential also. Encounters cannot happen if we are not there. We can provide an unself-conscious, comfort- able, unthreatening presence that puts people at ease. This re- quires a disregard of the public nature of the area, an ability to function effectively in the midst of a crowd.

The fourth ingredient is *readiness*. We must be alert to the moment, open to opportunity. I am reminded of Christ's appeal to his disciples in the Garden of Gethsemane. Disciples, I need you. I need you now, I need you close, I need you awake. They must have regretted missing a serendipitous moment with Jesus because of their unreadiness.

Serendipity can happen as we superimpose the internal model onto the external one (fig. 3). Serendipity is finding something valuable that we were not seeking, that we did not expect. It is being surprised by grace-filled moments. It is adventure.

These models open a place for the Spirit to enter and provide encounters that the patients and I treasure. While these principles are easily articulated, they are much more difficult for me to follow. But I believe that the Spirit blesses our intention, sen- sitivity, visibility, and readiness. Do not sleep through those mo- ments—they are precious.

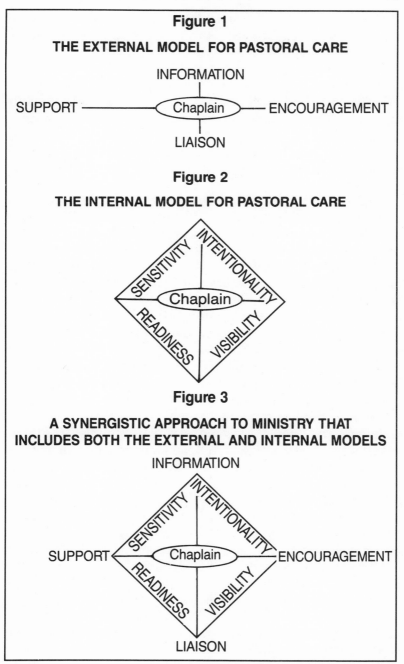

Figure 1

THE EXTERNAL MODEL FOR PASTORAL CARE

INFORMATION

SUPPORT — Chaplain — ENCOURAGEMENT

LIAISON

Figure 2

THE INTERNAL MODEL FOR PASTORAL CARE

SENSITIVITY INTENTIONALITY
Chaplain
READINESS VISIBILITY

Figure 3

A SYNERGISTIC APPROACH TO MINISTRY THAT INCLUDES BOTH THE EXTERNAL AND INTERNAL MODELS

INFORMATION

SENSITIVITY INTENTIONALITY
SUPPORT Chaplain ENCOURAGEMENT
READINESS VISIBILITY

LIAISON

V. Reflections on Ministry
By Sister Margaret Whooley

The patients I minister to are not only physically sick but are caught in the complex network of an institution, dealing with adjustments in life-style and schedules, and struggling with problems of housing and care for loved ones as well as their own care. The diversity of emotional and spiritual needs can be even greater than that of physical needs, ranging from optimistic trust in modern medicine to feelings of defeat in being dependent on others.

The families are greatly involved in their sick members' care, and patients share concern for the condition of each other. Most have heard much about diagnosis and prognosis and are sorting out the verbal and nonverbal communications they have received.

The chaplain ministers in this milieu with and through the health care team that recognizes his or her role as supportive for them as well as for the patients and families. He or she is called to deal with anxiety, fear, hostility, and alienation but also to focus on and affirm the human strengths in faith, trust, courage, and peace.

The ministry includes the effective presence of the chaplain, creative listening and waiting, offering perspective, responding to the need for prayer, Scripture, and sacrament, and compassion and healing through peace and vision.

In ministry I respond to requests and referrals, institution availability, the call within myself, and human interaction within God's creative presence. There is a challenge and there are questions. I wonder if I am willing, available, and vulnerable to risk fulfilling my part in the healing profession, to be a focus for sensitivity to the presence of the Divine Healer and to the uniqueness of individuals, to evoke the potential within persons to be part of their own healing, and to connect wounds with the wounds of all humanity and with the Suffering Servant of God. "What one person suffers, all suffer" (1 Cor. 12:36). How do I discern and encourage movements that can support and restore values of self-esteem and confidence? When and how do I initiate or facilitate help from other appropriate sources, such as the parish, social service, or advocacy staff?

A recent example of accumulated concern is a 54-year-old man who had become acutely ill without prior medical attention. His wife approached me about 9:00 A.M. showing shock and confusion. The experience was overwhelming to her. All the things that needed attention were welling up within her to the point that she saw medical care to be of no avail to her husband. (The doctors had told her the seriousness of his condition.) She asked me if I knew of hospice care. She expressed concern about her commitments for the day, contacting her family, waiting for reports, and other matters.

Then she spoke of her fear of losing her husband and added, "He hasn't been to church but now he is too weak." We talked about that and I said I would go see him. He was weak and saddened by his condition, but very much in touch with his faith.

As the hours passed, they both received the care and concern of the staff. Together they became more peaceful, more in touch with life and its fragility, more aware of their treasured memories and important life values. The patient died about 7:00 P.M., having been ministered to by a chaplain of his own faith. His wife had contacted their family's pastor during the day.

I see outpatient ministry as being where the need is, as healing relationships on individual, family, and institution levels. It is helping persons retreat from complex surroundings to discover their inner riches, often at times when all seems lost.

Notes

1. Henri Nouwen, *The Living Reminder* (New York: The Seabury Press, 1977), 44.
2. Ibid.

Chapter 4

THE CLINIC–PARISH CONNECTION

Ronald H. Sunderland

Seventeen years ago, when I began to inch my way toward the design and implementation of a training program to equip lay-people to play their full part in the pastoral ministry of the congregation, I approached the concept from my vantage point as a member of the clergy. Biblically, theologically, and historically, it was clear that pastoral ministry at the parish level required calling into ministry those members gifted with pastoral care skills. The centering of pastoral ministry exclusively in the clergy office was an aberration of the biblical message. What I discovered as soon as the issues were identified and explored was that lay-people had never been *un*involved in pastoral care in the congregation; their work had simply not been recognized as ministry, nor were they recognized as ministers in the fullest New Testament sense of *diakonoi*. While clergy had assumed the pastoral ministry function as belonging to the clergy office, church members were constantly involved in pastoral care of one another, and, of course, exercising their gifts beyond the congregation's bounds as surely as they did within them. The tragedy lay in the failure of their respective faith groups to recognize that pastoral care is intrinsically a *congregational*, not exclusively a *clergy*, task and that laypeople are constantly engaged in ministry.[1] This concept is fully validated in the Scriptures, and is receiving widespread support and taking shape nationally in lay training programs in congregations, such as my *Equipping Lay People for Ministry* design.[2]

One manifestation of the concept is apparent in outpatient ministry. Quietly and unostentatiously over the years, laypeople have accompanied members of their congregations to outpatient clinics, providing nurture and support, helping patients hear what physicians have imparted, crying or rejoicing with them, and standing by them as outpatient visit followed outpatient visit.

The ministry of St. Paul's United Methodist congregation, located adjacent to the Texas Medical Center in Houston, is a graphic illustration. Twenty-three years ago, the congregation purchased property adjacent to the church on which a block of apartments stood. Pursuing its vision of a ministry to patients and families using the facilities of the medical center, St. Paul's began to seek the assistance of other congregations to put the vacant apartments to their most effective use. First Christian Church in Pasadena, Texas, located 10 miles from the center, was one of the first congregations to participate in the program. The First Christian congregation paid the rent on one of the units and coordinated the use of the apartment by out-of-town patients who had been admitted for medical care as outpatients at hospitals in the medical center, or by families with members in the hospital.

Care for families accommodated in the units was provided by members of various participating congregations. The action of St. Paul's, long before McDonalds was inspired to replicate the program in the Ronald McDonald houses so familiar in larger cities, quickly inspired other versions of the concept. Dr. Joe Hightower, a member of Bering Drive Church of Christ and a Rice University faculty member, led a team of people in the initiation of a project that in 1989 consisted of 21 apartments (the goal is 37) available to outpatients and families of inpatients from other states and countries. Each person or family is offered pastoral support by laypeople who have made this their locus of ministry. South Main Baptist and Memorial Drive Presbyterian congregations each support similar programs, providing accommodation and pastoral care to patients and families using their facilities. The number of apartments available in Houston now exceeds 36, and the number is growing.

As professionals in ministry, we have tended to apply our concepts according to visions limited by our institutional identities. Thus, outpatient pastoral care has been narrowly interpreted to apply to those activities undertaken by department of pastoral care staffs within the confines of the institution itself; it was what occurred in the outpatient clinic. For example, what happened beyond the clinic when outpatients returned to their homes and congregations was not strictly the department's business. Frankly, our work was done when they walked out of the clinic or when we left the hospital after the day's work was over.

Now we are much more aware that all that is changing, and we must not so much adapt to the changes as participate in them, share in the structuring of change, and develop forms of ministry that are appropriate and effective in the changing environment of health care. This has special significance for pastoral care with outpatients.

First, we have acknowledged that life's boundaries for outpatients are not fixed at the elevator door or the front door of the hospital: the visit to the outpatient clinic was just one day out of the week. Second, this means that those people who carry the *primary* pastoral care responsibility for outpatients (family members, fellow members of congregations, and their ordained clergy) fulfil a much broader ministry than clinic chaplains. Third, this changing vision of institutional care including pastoral care opens up new areas of responsibility for institutional chaplains.

The Community (Not the Hospital) as the Locus for Patient Care

It may seem somewhat strange to confess that when we as staff chaplains began to explore the nature and scope of outpatient ministry, we began with the assumption that our investigation was restricted to the geographic boundaries of our respective clinics. It certainly was naive on our part, and indicates how easily professionals can become accustomed to limiting their boundaries to their work settings. However, once the boundaries were dissolved we could see patients in *their* locations, which were not the hospitals but their communities. A patient's hospital visit absorbed a few hours (although all too often that became an entire day), but home and other responsibilities and relationships await- ed them. Some health care professionals too glibly refer to whol- istic medicine but confine that term to the involvement of a multidisciplinary team in the hospital segment of the patient's life. Both Holst and Anderson remind us in their essays that, among their other roles, chaplains are called to exercise a pro- phetic function within their institutions and within their faith groups. This must apply within the outpatient clinic programs in our hospitals where medical care normally depends on the multidisciplinary team, to which the patient's pastor might, in some cases, make a significant contribution. I believe we have not challenged medical or nursing staffs with sufficient vigor to view patients as members of families and communities, and often of congregations. Nor have we taken with sufficient seriousness the opportunities that exist to establish links between the limited pastoral ministry the institution can offer and the broader min- istry that encompasses the patient's life beyond the hospital. The question is what steps we may take to facilitate conversations between the hospital and the parish.

The Congregation as the Locus for Ministry

One of our tasks—and one of the important reasons for out- patient pastoral ministry—is to ensure that patients are perceived as people whose location is not the hospital but the community. Chaplains also bear the responsibility of taking the initiative to invite patients' pastors to see the hospital as the extension of their care of their own members. Parish clergy fulfill a much more intensive pastoral function than chaplains can in their brief patient encounters. Chaplains must acknowledge that a primary objective of their ministry should include the support of patients' congre- gations where most of their pastoral support is located. The support of the patients' primary pastoral caregivers, lay and or- dained, should be high on the chaplain's list of priorities. Chap- lains should support them rather than regard them as mere adjuncts of their own services. Chaplains thus find the fulfillment of ministry in the servant role demanded by the scriptures.

Strengthening the Clinic-Parish Connection

There ought now to be a much clearer understanding that a closer working and educational relationship between clinic chaplains and parish clergy is long overdue. The first thought among the M. D. Anderson Cancer Center staff was to capitalize on our experience with part-time (extended-quarter) C.P.E. programs; perhaps we might recruit pastors and selected laypeople to participate in a 10-hour-a-week program, assigning them to one of the hospital's 30 outpatient clinics. This notion was put on hold until the staff chaplains were more thoroughly versed in the structuring of clinic ministry. As we investigated this, new concerns emerged: Did the particular characteristics of clinic medical and nursing care require a continuous presence of the chaplain, not only once a day, but several times each day? If so, how many clinics could one person oversee, and could a clinic's pastoral ministry needs be served by an extended-quarter student?

We have concluded tentatively that outpatient ministry is, in fact, labor intensive. If chaplains are to make a meaningful effort in clinic ministry, they must be present in the clinic for some portion of each day. We quickly became aware that each clinic functions as an integrated team, especially in hospitals like M. D. Anderson, where experimental drugs are constantly being tested and physicians, pathologists, nurses, social workers, laboratory technicians, and others are all involved in monitoring patients. The chaplain either remains an outsider to the group or seeks to be fully a part of the program. Herbert Anderson calls chaplains to fulfill a prophetic role in the hospital and to be aware of their unique "outsider" role. Yet chaplains cannot gain the confidence of other staff members and earn the right to challenge nursing or medical practices unless they and their work are known and respected. The physical presence of the chaplain, committing time each day to the clinic patients and the staff members who attend them, is of paramount importance.

On this basis, we decided to develop effective ministries in a limited number of clinics and to defer the introduction of part-time personnel. Was there any place for the involvement of members of congregations in clinic ministry? The strong desire expressed by clergy staff of St. Paul's United Methodist Church to exercise a ministry in the medical center suggested the first direction in which to proceed.

St. Paul's, as one of the first United Methodist congregations in the city to develop lay pastoral care ministry under supervision, was linked through the hospital's pastoral care department with an out-of-state outpatient and her family. Members of the pastoral care team provided social support to the family as did members of a United Methodist congregation in their family's home city. The visitors were invited to worship at St. Paul's during the stay in Houston. Meals and other outings were shared. A member of Memorial Drive Presbyterian Church likewise befriended an outpatient who was receiving medical care in one of our clinics and staying in one of that congregation's medical center apartments. He was alone in Houston, his wife having returned to their home to continue care of their family. The pastoral support rendered by this lay ministry made his stay in Houston and consequent separation from his family more bearable. Faith Lutheran Church, also close to the medical center and with three apartments, provided accommodation to a Southern Baptist family and supported the patient and his wife through an extensive period of outpatient care that ended with the patient's death.

The Unspoken Question

At many points in our individual, family, and corporate lives, questions lie like land mines that we are hesitant to ask and hope others will not ask. The problem resides in the dilemmas implicit in our questions: if they are asked publicly, they must be addressed. If left unasked, they somehow may go away—a clear case of denial. Herbert Anderson has asked the question directly: Is there a role for pastoral ministry in the clinic? My hunch is that our staff chaplain committee on outpatient ministry at M. D. Anderson Cancer Center was a little afraid of this question. Do we answer "yes" merely to justify our place in the sun? When we finally asked the question of ourselves, we were able to acknowledge that we believe there is, in fact, an essential role for chaplains. We trusted our intuitions because they were supported by our clinical experience. We may have been uncertain just how to fulfill our ministry, but that the ministry was needed became a matter of certainty.

The problems lie in other directions. First, we concluded that clinic ministry is sufficiently different from inpatient pastoral care, requiring a significant level of training, experience, and time commitment as to exclude the assignment of first-year student chaplains to clinics. More experienced chaplains may be assigned, provided that the clinic assignment is a primary function. Second, we concluded that commitment to clinic ministry by a department of pastoral care cannot be for appearance's sake, a sort of public relations gesture. Third, the opportunities and needs for ministry far outstripped our capacities to meet them. In common with hospitals nationwide, limited funding of chaplaincy services will restrict our ability to provide comprehensive coverage of all the institution's facilities as far into the future as we can see. Hence, choices must be made concerning which areas our limited means can serve. This conclusion was reinforced by our conviction that the time we make available to clinics must be quality time, concentrated in not more than two areas, if we were to do more than just walk through waiting areas and chat with a few people. Fourth, although I believe the term *burnout* is ambiguous and its relationship to unrecognized and therefore unresolved grief has not been adequately explored, it is the most commonly recognized warning to personnel who work in situations in which ambivalence and stress are commonplace. Clinic chaplains will do well to ensure that they have access to a solid support system of peer support and counseling.

If one thinks in terms of a master plan for the development of clinic ministry, the program of matching congregations with families in need of support as outlined above is an appealing starting point. This assumes it incorporates oversight of the lay pastoral care team's ministry. The second step, if the department has a working relationship with a number of participating congregations, would be to select a number of clergy and lay "students" from the parish programs for recruitment to a part-time in-house education program involving assignment of the student group to a limited number of clinics, and ministering under intensive oversight.

Are we any further advanced than when we began to assess the effectiveness of our existing outpatient ministry and to project what would be required of us if we were to commit to that ministry the effort it both needed and deserved? Certainly, we understand much more clearly the nature and scope of the opportunity we confront. We know also that in the brief period during which we have made a concerted attempt to be present in our clinics and to become acquainted with our respective fellow staff members, our presence was affirmed and staff looked to us for the same commitment they were making themselves. From the responses of patients with whom we have spent "quality time," we are sure that patients and their family members need and value our ministry.

All that is affirming. But the most important insight we have gained is that we have only just begun our work. Ahead of us lie the tasks of testing various models for extending outpatient pastoral care. We must find ways to invite parish clergy and the congregations to which they minister to help us link our ministry with theirs, remembering that hospital-based pastoral care is complementary to their primary base of ministry in the congregation.

If we have "discovered" any new insights from our reflections on our clinic ministries, they are, first, that we have established firmly our conviction that the chaplain has an important role to fill in the clinics. This is affirmed both by our own day-by-day experiences and by the urgency with which we have been welcomed by clinic personnel.

Second, I believe that we are on the way to establishing that the outpatient clinic is an appropriate setting for continuing pastoral education for ordained and laypeople from congregations. If our tentative conclusion is valid, we ought to draw up plans to introduce a model with a carefully designed plan to formulate the program and to monitor its implementation under the oversight of a task force drawn from hospital services (medical, nursing, social service) that also includes lay and clergy members of congregations.

Third, I believe it is essential that clinic chaplains commit themselves to regular peer support and planning sessions as a departmental function. An individual staff chaplain without other chaplain staff support in a smaller institution could acquire similar peer support by meeting with other clinic staff, for example, social workers or nurses.

The clinic chaplains at the Cancer Center do not claim to have identified all the assets or liabilities that assist or inhibit our clinic ministries. We have taken our first, uncertain steps. Now we must learn to walk. We are now aware that we have company and are not alone in either recognizing the importance of our ministry or our own private anxieties about being present in the clinics. We hope other chaplains will participate in this venture by sharing their experiences and encourage them to do so through pastoral care journals and other publications.

Notes

1. Ronald H. Sunderland, "Lay Pastoral Care," in *Primary Pastoral Care* (Atlanta: Journal of Pastoral Care Publications, Inc. 1990), 65–82.

2. Sunderland, *Equipping Laypeople for Minstry* (Houston: ELM, Inc., 1983).

Chapter 5

A MINISTRY OF OPENNESS

Betty Adam

In 1987 the University of Texas M. D. Anderson Cancer Center in Houston, Texas, added a 10-story clinic building to its sprawling complex. The addition was especially remarkable, for it was not just another hospital added to the Texas Medical Center. The building was an outpatient facility. Its massiveness signaled that the age of outpatient care had arrived.

The trend toward outpatient care in the medical community has altered the work of the chaplain. Today, the majority of patients at the M. D. Anderson Cancer Center are outpatients. Though hospital beds are still occupied, and chaplains are regularly assigned to specific floors within the hospital, there are in addition an average of 1,500 daily appointments within the clinic building. Some of the outpatients coming in for appointments are healthy, some are very sick, and others are dying. It must be acknowledged that many need pastoral care. The age of outpatient ministry has arrived.

How are those in need of pastoral care to be located within the massive structure? How is pastoral care in the clinic to get its start? Is this a new kind of ministry? Are there any real differences between outpatient ministry and inpatient ministry?

These were some of the questions asked at the Anderson Center by a group of six chaplains who were particularly interested in developing outpatient pastoral care. The group met on a bi-monthly basis to explore their experiences and investigate this seemingly new kind of ministry. In January 1989 they hosted a National Conference on Outpatient Ministry with the College of Chaplains as a response to this new challenge in ministry. This paper is an extension of the presentation I gave at that conference.

The most widely accepted model for the ministry of hospital chaplains has been an inclusive one that assumes every patient will receive a visit from a staff member. In some larger hospitals, where denominational chaplains are appointed as staff members, the task is eased somewhat by the assumption that denominational chaplains will look after their respective patients. Some hospitals adopt the policy that all new patients will be visited within 24 hours of admission. This attempt to provide comprehensive coverage is unworkable in outpatient clinics; the number of patients is too great.

But by what criteria is the range of coverage narrowed? The pastoral care staff may have difficulty deciding which of the many clinics can be covered, and then some selection process may be needed within each clinic. For example, should patient visits be made according to priorities, patients in the most severe stages of illness or only on referral from another staff member? Is it best to make initial contact with new patients, tell them about the chaplaincy service, try to assess their level of need, and then try to match the chaplain's time in the clinic with return visits by those patients? Is denominational matching of chaplains and patients practical in the outpatient clinic?

It might be thought that priority should be given to the new patients in a manner similar to that adopted by social workers; that is, seeing each patient on admission, receiving referrals from other staff members, and following them through the course of their clinic care. However, if the chaplain's work involves entering the patient's world, hearing his or her story, or helping sort out treatment possibilities, the right moment for ministry may not coincide with the patient's first clinic visit. New patients may not be ready to tell their stories, be able to let others into their worlds, or be aware of the possible courses and options for treatment and their need to discuss them.

If denominational chaplains are able to acquire the names of clinic patients by religious preference it might be thought that priority for contacting certain patients over others might be given by denomination or religious tradition. However, ministry in outpatient clinics may be overwhelming for many religious groups; efforts to locate patients and schedule appointments coinciding with return visits may be impractical unless the chaplain has assistance from a team of lay volunteers.

Moreover, there is a broad diversity among outpatients sitting in clinic waiting areas. Some are new patients, perhaps undergoing diagnostic workups, while others may have been in the system for many years. They may range from people present for a semiannual checkup confirming continuing satisfactory progress to others in deep crisis, perhaps facing the news that there is nothing further that the hospital can offer them.

Clinic ministry is overwhelming in terms of numbers and needs, and with respect to space and time limits. If it is impractical to provide comprehensive coverage or categorize patients in order to decide whom to visit, is there a "nonsystematic" model that is more applicable? Does one start each day by walking through the clinic and introducing oneself at random to waiting patients, hoping that spontaneous encounters will lead to ministry?

While chaplains receive referrals from the clinic personnel that set their agenda in reference to specific patients or their families, I believe general clinic ministry is bound to follow this open or nonsystematic model. When this occurs, there is no agenda other than being present and responsive to perceived needs. To use John Macquarrie's language, ministers "enable" or "empower" by their very presence.[1] Mother Teresa states that neither she nor her sisters had preconceived ideas about how to go about their work on the streets of Calcutta; they started their ministry when the suffering of people called them. God showed them what to do, and they went where God led and where there was need.[2]

By using this model, chaplains learn to be present in the clinic, both physically and spiritually, particularly in the waiting areas. Visibility is critical. There is a certain boldness in walking up and introducing oneself to a seated person. With no list to follow, no referral to be answered, no summons to "be here" and help in some specific manner, what remains is a sea of people and the spontaneous encounter that is its own fulfillment. The human contact, the existential moment that opens up and empowers—that is clinic ministry quintessentially.

In responding through this model, chaplains learn to be open, not closed off, by personal defenses, mocking burnout, and threatening fears. They learn to open out their fields of accessibility, to relinquish their need for ministry by steps or categories, and to risk openness to others. Clinics embrace a broad cross-section of people, and the same breadth is evident in the diversity of needs, and therefore the range of opportunities they present to chaplains. Chaplains constantly need to be open to the stranger and to be inclusive in their ministry; perhaps, with real openness, there are no strangers. From this perspective, openness means accepting the gift of openness to God's presence, mystery, and control. It means speaking freely to God under the love commandment, questioning the mystery of suffering that opens up in the light of God's presence, going beyond the last too-easily thought out answer or conclusion, wherever the patient or other person needs to venture. Venturing into areas where hopes and despairs mingle and where the opportunity for soul to meet soul is always present means developing the open self in moments that transcend finitude.

It also means to choose freely the responsibility of living in the presence of God, and to "open onto" the world. In Paul Ricouer's words, it is an opening out onto, not a presence to the self closed in on itself.[3] Here is intentionality beyond the self, an accepted call, a contemplation, and a prayer. For the person to whom the chaplain ministers, it is the relief of being heard and perhaps understood, a satisfying dialogue bearing the promise of healing, a tapping of resources of grace. Perhaps it is a discovery of his or her own open self which, as Karl Rahner stated, is already there as a supernatural existential.[4] Openness is a gift that links us to God. God is an open presence, and our connection to God is real when we present ourselves openly to others.

On what grounds is this model offered to clinic ministers? Furthermore, what does it mean theologically to suggest that a minister be open or that people be open to God's openness? What is the nature of the open self? How does this model fit within the Christian understanding of God's creation and God's redemption of the world?

Recently openness has been given value in family communication. It has captured a highlight in the theology of dialogue, and contemporary theologians have used the imagery of openness and narrowness, or of openness and closure, in epistemological and anthropological discussions. The popular concept of openness, according to Alan Bloom, is that which is ascribed to "progressive" and "forward-looking" persons without an ideology and value system, those asserting cultural relativism.[5]

However, the openness I refer to runs counter to Bloom's popular concept. In this model openness is grounded in the biblical notion. Open persons choose an absolute reference point, that of a specific spiritual object as understood within the Christian tradition; they choose an ideology and a value system. Karl Rahner's terminology of Jesus as "absolute Savior" is particularly applicable, the term referring to the incarnation as "the necessary and permanent beginning of the divinization of the world as a whole."[6] It is a Rahnerian view that with the birth and death of the historical person, Jesus of Nazareth, the highest moment of God's openness is marked, a moment bestowing a grace for the salvation of the whole world. By reference to this ultimate event Christians exercise their supreme possibility of saying yes to God's openness, and by reference to this absolute Savior their inward life and value system develop most fully. The open self, as defined here, cuts across all relativized frameworks and recognizes its absolute dependence upon God and its need for redemption in a world disordered by evil. It is precisely in coming to recognize one's own openness to the self-communication of God in Christ and in the ensuing development of a value system that one becomes open to others.

The key term for understanding the concept of openness is the Greek noun *parrhesia*. *Parrhesia* may be translated as "openness," but most often in the Revised Standard Version it is rendered "boldness," and in an extended sense, as "confidence" and "joyfulness." The use of the term in the New Testament is thoroughly discussed by Schlier in *The Theological Dictionary of the New Testament*.[7]

In the New Testament *parrhesia* has connections with ministry. In the Gospel of John, *parrhesia* is linked to the public ministry of Jesus, and according to Schlier "has a place in the Johannine dialectic of the revelation of Jesus."[8] A mark of Jesus as revealer is that he works publicly, or openly: his society is not a sect, and his preaching is not a secret doctrine. However, in a sense his *parrhesia* is concealed. He speaks in parables, rather than openly. Moreover, his *parrhesia* (if *parrhesia* can be translated as "manifestation" or "revelation," as Schlier suggests) is concealed from the disciples until his ascension and the coming of the Paraclete; that is, the *parrhesia* of Jesus is limited until the coming of the risen Lord in the Spirit.[9] *Parrhesia*, then, suggests the openness, or self-revelation, of God in Jesus.

Elsewhere in the Johannine corpus, *parrhesia* is used for human access or openness to God. First John suggests that if one's conscience is clear, he or she stands with *parrhesia* to God. Specifically, a clear conscience results from believing in Jesus as the Christ and the keeping of his love commandments. Furthermore, openness to God is given with the presence of the Spirit in us. *Parrhesia* to God is found where God indwells in those who keep the commandments of Jesus, and it finds expression in prayer to God, which God hears. Theologically, a concept of the open self may be developed from this biblical perspective. Christians would seek to develop the open self, which is opposed to shame and guilt, and fears no punishment. *Parrhesia* is a reflection of the fullness of the love of God in us.[10]

In the book of Acts, *parrhesia* is used with reference to the Christian's openness to others, and it is a gift of the Spirit to be used in ministry to the public. The public is hostile, so *parrhesia* may be rendered as candor or boldness. It is a risk. For example, the *parrhesia* of Peter and John in Acts 4:13 surprises the Jewish authorities who know that the apostles are not trained in rhetorical ability. Because the Lord gives *parrhesia* to his servants, their power is different than the power of those trained by human leaders.[11]

Elsewhere in the Pauline corpus, Paul speaks of *parrhesia* in a general context of ministers of the new covenant. In that context Paul combines openness to God and openness to others. It also includes openness to the gospel.[12] In 2 Cor. 3:4-18 Paul implies that ministers of the new covenant who have lifted their faces uncovered to God also turn uncovered to other human beings. In an extended sense, according to Schlier, openness suggests "affection" to others and a close association with *exousia* (right or power).[13] It is nonconcealment and a reflection of the glory of the Lord. Christ is the agent of this openness. The person in Christ finds freedom toward God and can approach God with confidence.[14]

In Hebrews, according to Schlier, *parrhesia* connotes a distinctive mode of being on the part of the Christian. As E. Käsemann has suggested, *parrhesia* has an objective character.[15] One has it, not as a subjective attitude, but as an appropriation of something already there. One keeps it by faith in the promise. Openness is worked out in a life that has entered into openness. Hebrews 3:6 asks that we hold fast to *parrhesia*, which is a freedom of access to God, an authority to enter the sanctuary, an openness to the new and living way that Jesus has restored. The saving work of Jesus has created *parrhesia* and made its fulfillment possible.[16]

This model of openness draws upon the epistemology of God and the ontological structures of the human being as analyzed in contemporary theology, particularly in the works of John Macquarrie, Karl Rahner, and Paul Ricoeur. It is Macquarrie who uses the concept most specifically and clearly. He defines "to exist" as "to have an openness," openness being a gift in the epistemology of God and a clue to the mysterious affinity of God and human beings. Macquarrie suggests that God opens himself into creation in self-giving and in communication; he brings into being. He also enables creatures to be and empowers them to "let-be." Just as God opens himself into creation and has "letting-be" as his essence, so human beings are truly themselves and realize themselves most freely when they can let be, or have an openness in responsibility, in creativity, and in love. Macquarrie conceives of the *imago Dei* as an openness conceptualized in terms of a potentiality that is given to people into which they can move upward and outward. In this way creaturely being is taken up into Holy Being.[17]

Karl Rahner speaks of the "essential openness" of persons.[18] For Rahner, openness is an expression of what can be originally experienced within the depths of existence. Spirit is a valid category and human beings are constituted spiritually by a basic openness to the unlimited expanse of reality. That human beings are open to God is a way of saying that they are beings of transcendence to the Holy. As human beings we are structured with a basic openness to God that is prior to the exercise of our freedom to accept or reject God. Closure of this openness takes place when a person says no.

Rahner argues that what opens before persons in transcendental experience is not something subject to their own power: what opens up is experienced as something established by another. It is not self-generated but is the work of that to which people are open, namely, being in an absolute sense. Here there is a movement of hope and the desire to reach out, a movement toward liberating freedom and responsibility. This openness, or movement to transcendence, is the infinite horizon of Being making itself manifest. Whenever we experience ourselves as questioning and as open to something ineffable, we cannot understand ourselves as absolute subjects but only in the sense of one receiving Being, ultimately in the sense of grace. Thus openness is a movement of grace, where grace means a freedom given by God for human beings to move beyond their finitude and contingency.[19]

Paul Ricoeur develops his understanding of the a priori structures of the human subject out of humanity's knowledge relation to the world. When he shifts attention from the object to the body to whom it appears, it is "openness onto the world" that he finds characteristic. For Ricoeur this openness is a finite one. By examining receptivity, openness is seen to be limited in its perspective; every view of the world is a point of view. And yet it is the nature of human finitude that it can experience itself only on the condition that there be a "view-on" finitude, a dominating look that has already begun to transgress finitude; that is, the act by which we become aware of point of view reveals an elementary connection between an experience of infinitude and a movement transgressing this finitude.

In exploring the dialectic between the finite and the infinite in human beings, Ricoeur is drawn to the image of openness because it suggests the mixture of point of view and meaning that he has discovered; point of view is a narrowness of humanity's openness, but the image of openness suggests something beyond this perspective. Openness accounts for the transgression of point of view and for humanity's not being enclosed within each silhouette of perspective. Openness suggests that human beings have access to a space of expressibility. For Ricoeur perspective and transgression are two poles of a single function of openness and the image of openness captures the mixture of humanity's ability to synthesize in the imagination presence and meaning.[20]

This paper argues for moments in our daily experience that transcend our finite perspective. We draw our energies and resources for Christian creative living from these transcendent moments. As Ricoeur has suggested, in these moments there is a feeling of expansiveness and extension beyond the mere self enclosed in on itself and an openness out to God and to others.

Human persons are always developing in their openness. They open out beyond themselves, push out from under the oppressive closures of their own personal history and cultural environment, and move more and more into God's light. The open self is a social self responding to God and community, a dynamic self full of change and development seeking more reality.

As we learn to be open, inclusive, and accessible, our ministry with outpatients is transformed. We are saying "yes" to God's openness and in doing so, we convey God's love and healing presence. Inclusivity in this context is not statistical, having less to do with comprehensiveness than with accessibility to opportunity. A willingness to listen and respond to expressed needs, a making contact with God's will and word, a commitment to move into the intimacy of the presented moments work together for what I believe is appropriate in the clinic context, despite numbers and overwhelming odds.

Notes

1. John Macquarrie, *Principles of Christian Theology* (New York: Charles Scribner's Sons, 1977), 113, 230.

2. Eileen Egan, *Such a Vision of the Street* (Garden City, N.Y.: Doubleday and Co., Inc., 1985), 44.

3. Paul Ricoeur, *Fallible Man* (New York: Fordham Univ. Press, 1986), 19.

4. Karl Rahner, *Foundations of Christian Faith* (New York: Crossroad, 1982), 126.

5. Alan Bloom, *The Closing of the American Mind* (New York: Simon & Schuster, 1987), 25–43.

6. Rahner, *Foundations*, 181, 193–95.

7. Gerhard Kittel, ed., *The Theological Dictionary of the New Testament* (Grand Rapids: Wm. B. Eerdmans, 1964), 871–84.

8. Kittel, 879.

9. Ibid., 880–81.

10. Ibid., 881–82.

11. Ibid., 882.

12. Ibid., 883.

13. Ibid.

14. Ibid.

15. Ibid., 884.

16. Ibid.

17. Macquarrie, *Principles*, 113–14.

18. Rahner, *Foundations*, 19–20, 37–38, 100–1.

19. Rahner, 34–35.

20. Ricoeur, *Fallible*, 19–26, 37–40.

Chapter 6

COMMUNITY HEALTH CENTER MINISTRY

Lorna Jean T. Miller

One setting for outpatient ministry is community health centers. For 15 years the chaplaincy department of the Harris County Hospital District has been developing priorities and providing care for health center patients, their families, and the employees working with them.

The Harris County Hospital District serves medically indigent people of Houston, Texas, and surrounding communities with 3 hospitals and 11 community health centers. The centers offer the professional services of adult and pediatric physicians, nurses, chaplains, nutritionists, and social workers. Laboratories, X rays, and pharmacies are also available on site. These centers average 2,000 to 4,000 patient visits per center per month. During 1988, the Harris County Hospital District had a total of 98,850 emergency center visits, and 597,590 outpatient visits. There were 258,491 visits in the Community Health Program.

The chaplaincy department provides coverage at eight of these centers one day per week: one full-time staff chaplain covers five centers and a part-time chaplain covers the other three. Currently a chaplain intern is also serving at one of these centers eight hours a week. In our hospital district, the work of the chaplain is directed from a districtwide office and coordinated with the Community Health Program administrator and the director and medical director of each center.

As chaplains, our number-one priority is the patients. This can be seen in the following statement: "The philosophy of the department is based on the innate value of the human person and on the enhancement of his/her hopes for recovering and/or maintaining health through being served by the total health care team. This is a wholistic approach to the care of the patient in which the interaction of spiritual and faith responses is seen as essential to the administration of physical remedies" (Departmental Philosophy excerpt, 1982). We are about the ministry of healing, sustaining, and guiding as participating members of the health care team. The chaplain takes an approach to pastoral care that encompasses the physical, psychological, and spiritual dimensions necessary to the patients' total health care.

In medical literature it is well documented that stress and anxiety are contributing factors in many disease processes. The focus of pastoral listening and care is not so much in relieving the problems in peoples' lives but in transmitting a positive viewpoint and developing coping skills using their spiritual gifts for living more fully in the present situation. "I have come that you might have life—life in its fullness" (John 10:10b paraphrase).

The services of chaplaincy departments in community health centers are supportive pastoral listening for adults and children, consultation with other members of the health care team, referral to community agencies for psychotherapy or crisis support groups, and referral to and consultation with community clergy and churches of the patients' religious backgrounds.

Patients are scheduled to see chaplains by the computerized appointment system used for the other professional providers and services. They may also be sent by direct referral from another provider on the day that a chaplain is in the center. The chaplain makes rounds in the various waiting areas; some patients request to see him or her. The chaplain has an office area in each center; sometimes this space is private and sometimes it is shared.

Appointed patient visits are briefly documented in the medical record. A large file card that records in more detail pertinent data about the patient and the pastoral encounter is kept for each patient. The chaplaincy department keeps daily reports listing the name of the patient, the type of visit, and significant issues raised in that visit.

The ministry is very much a marketplace ministry as the chaplain moves about in open waiting areas, noticing a facial expression, a frequent visitor, or the tone of a conversation between nurse and patient. It is to be ready for the doctor's request, "Chaplain, I have a woman in my office who. . . ." This is a ministry like Jesus' ministry: on the move, responding to situations as they arise. At first this style of ministry may feel uncomfortable to one familiar with the more traditional bedside ministry in the inpatient setting.

Community health center chaplains need to be outgoing and capable of initiating a number of new relationships every day. Being creative, faithful, and flexible enough to move with the hour-by-hour flow of business also helps outpatient chaplains. We have to put patients and others at ease by affirming and supporting their measure of health and wholeness. We have one-time encounters with some and ongoing relationships that develop over months or years with others.

Some chaplains fear that the issues of privacy and confidentiality will be threatened in such a "marketplace" setting. But we need to let our patients also be our teachers. Remember that the God who gives us peace and makes us holy in every way keeps our whole being—spirit, soul, and body—free from every fault at the coming of our Lord Jesus Christ. He who calls us will do it because he is faithful (see 1 Thess. 5:23-24). We are called to this ministry, and its dimensions will develop as we respond to this call.

In community health centers, we may listen to a man who is out of work and struggling with a newly imposed sense of exile, pray with a woman who lived under bridges in Houston during her childhood and is now approaching three years of sobriety, talk with a woman making progress on a weight-loss plan, or counsel a woman and her teenage son who are grieving the death of the family's one-month-old baby. Adults, children, families are our clients. We listen to a boy who has never met his father but is happy to have been accepted into the Big Brothers program and a teenage refugee from El Salvador who is learning to sing a new song in a strange land.

The elderly are frequent visitors to our health centers. We may be called on to help them because they have not developed adequate faith resources and coping skills. For example, a stillbirth or a parent's death may not have been sufficiently grieved; and angers, hurts, or life events may not have been fully celebrated or forgiven. A man described a recent assault in his own home; an elderly woman brought her scrapbook of 50 years of a women's church group's work. Family photos are sometimes shared during initial assessment, or later when we discuss particular family members. Sometimes a phone visit takes the place of a face-to-face conversation with those who are homebound either because of their own limitations or because they have to stay home to care for an ill family member. Anniversaries are sometimes the occasions for a phone call following a death or other life-changing event.

Worship and prayer also have a place in community health center chaplaincy. Worship happens in the reading of Scripture, singing of a hymn with someone no longer able to sing in a choir, acting out a parable with a child, or discussing a prayer's significance followed by the prayer itself. Prayer life may be supported in small groups, and caregivers can include prayer in the celebration of significant occasions.

Community health center ministry is a ministry on the move. It is a ministry of faith and fellowship. At our central office in Ben Taub General Hospital, a banner summarizes our care and concern for the poor and the health center outpatient as part of that population. Paraphrasing Matt. 25:37-40, it says: " 'Lord, when did we see you hungry or thirsty, a stranger or naked, sick or in prison? Lord, when?' 'Whenever you did it for one of my brothers or sisters *here*, you did it for me.' "

Chapter 7

MINISTRY TO PERSONS WITH AIDS

Mary Grace

I wish to address the prophetic role of chaplains in relation to outpatient care for people living with AIDS and to chaplains' healing ministries with them. Two consequences of HIV progressive disease add to the difficulties people with AIDS face when they are hospitalized. First, the institutionalization of hospitals inevitably results in depersonalizing patient care, and as a result AIDS patients suffer more than most. Second, the intraphysic stresses of this infection are catastrophic and enervating.

Depersonalization of Patient Care

People are too often seen in terms of numbers and dollars. Individuals may feel lost in an institution that often seems impervious to the needs of patients. Chaplains also need to be aware that AIDS patients generally have carried HIV infection in its latent form for 5 to 10 years prior to entering the hospital. Their hospital stays are often prolonged and pain-filled. Countless needle-sticks, bronchoscopies, lumbar punctures, bilateral bone marrow biopsies, and highly toxic experimental drugs are routine. All too often the panic and frustration felt by clinic staff as they treat a disease assumed to be fatal translates into negative behavior patterns at the bedside. Patients may be regarded as experimental subjects. Physicians making rounds may discuss patients in the third-person singular and make therapeutic decisions and order diagnostic procedures without explanation.

Further difficulties arise from the fact that government guidelines that authorize financial assistance to persons with AIDS or with diseases attributable to AIDS lag pitifully behind the burgeoning mutation of infections considered to be HIV-related. Thus the government becomes another institution that adds to the process of dehumanization, leaves the financial support of people with AIDS in jeopardy, and further erodes self-esteem when patients can no longer work.

The second factor that accentuates the process of dehumanization is the tacit message that stems from deeply held convictions that have been drawn from the Deuteronomic theodicy. Many people believe God punishes evil and rewards good. I think persons with AIDS are abandoned not because of fear of contracting HIV infection but from fear of attracting God's retribution by association with them. For example, it is manifested when hospital staff gown, glove, and mask before taking blood pressures or temperatures, or delivering meal trays. It is also apparent when clergy administer a blessing from the doorway, but do not enter the room to touch patients, or when visiting church members leave pamphlets that refer to hellfire and damnation, but not of reconciliation. It is most painfully apparent when family members fail to visit patients.

I have painted an all-too-typical scenario of people with AIDS who begin the journey toward ill-health hidden from others because of the acute psychosocial pain of HIV-positive diagnosis, and who experience an intense sense of vulnerability with hospitalization. In this context, it is important to recognize that preparation for outpatient care must begin with the first in-hospital admission. This is particularly important with respect to pastoral ministry. If this does not receive attention, it is likely that we will lose them on discharge. Because people with AIDS struggle continuously with shame, loss of self-esteem, worthlessness, depression, and denial, they are forced into "deep cover."

As an example, let me describe my own experience. In June 1988 I was contacted by the president of the San Antonio AIDS Foundation. At the time I was responsible for the ministry to people with AIDS in the Baptist Memorial Hospital. I was asked to establish a full-time ministry to clients of the foundation, including care for clients when in the hospital. It was necessary to establish how I would relate to in-hospital pastoral staffs. Would learning opportunities for clinical pastoral students be inhibited if I provided primary pastoral ministry to this patient population? I approached my ministry from the perspective of a parish priest responsible to visit parishioners, a role well recognized by hospital staff. Second, I maintained my relationship with staff and students by providing several didactic and interpersonal skills seminars on the subject of caring for people with AIDS.

As chaplain to the San Antonio AIDS foundation, my primary responsibilities were to establish strong supportive pastoral relationships with patients while they were in the hospital; to produce a mutually negotiated care plan for outpatient care and follow-up with the patients; and to monitor and supervise care partnerships between individual patients and local congregations. During the past several months, relationships of trust have been established with patients so that outpatient care is now instituted at the beginning of the disease process. People with HIV positive diagnosis, newly diagnosed, are requesting counseling and access to support groups. The outpatient caseload of people requesting support prior to their first hospitalization is growing. Furthermore, our requests for care partners, or buddies, is growing faster than we can enroll and train laity.

The training of care partners differs from other buddy training programs that make no reference to pastoral care and theological integration. The San Antonio program begins on a theological foundation of hope and reconciliation. It avoids any reference to aggressive evangelical demands upon patients. In the nine years in which I have been concerned with ministry to people with AIDS, I have yet to encounter an AIDS patient who is not dealing at some level with remorse and sadness at the folly of past behavior recognized as part of the human condition. To demand that people with AIDS have a clear, consistent theology is to arrive fully loaded with our own agenda. To be able to hunker down and wait with a compassionate, listening heart initiates the pastoral ministry of reconciliation that leads to hope.

Intraphysic Stresses

The second problem for people with AIDS arises from patients' intraphysic struggles with the disease and the psychosocial issues that seem to engulf them. Repeatedly I see desperation, displacement, and disequilibrium. The sense of desperation experienced by people with AIDS is manifested in an overwhelming anxiety and need to employ extreme measures in an attempt to escape the bitterness of frustration. Everyday life takes on urgency with the loss of social, professional, and financial stability. In just four months a patient may lose a well-paying job with its accompanying comfortable, middle-class perquisites, and face food stamps along with welfare applications. Patients watch lovers, friends, and acquaintances die, and are overcome with the inevitability of their own deaths. They realize there may be little time for extended therapy. Denial becomes the companion of substance abuse. In fact, we now routinely treat alcoholism and drug addiction side by side with HIV infection.

People living with AIDS may become refugees in their own communities. Families of origin often withdraw support. Sons and daughters often leave home to ease the pain of expected rejection. Family systems are torn asunder, with all sharing the humiliation of social branding. They feel like lepers. The socially displaced join others like themselves and become a social enclave under the guise of community.

Disequilibrium among people with AIDS is reflected in the radical fluctuations of emotional responses to everyday life that anyone in the bereavement process encounters. Not only are bodily functions and systems out of balance, but the mind and spirit as well. The emotional roller coaster of AIDS engenders its own fear, and heightened fear spawns loss of control and powerlessness.

Patients beset with such catastrophic stress may experience what I call AIDS psychosis. Physicians are seeing this more frequently. These psychotic episodes are neither a result of neuropathy nor drugs. Let me give you an example.

Bob was looking forward to being discharged from the hospital after treatment for Kaposi's sarcoma. He had been in the hospital for 61 days. He had left his home in Dallas when he was diagnosed with HIV infection and moved to San Antonio, where he alternately lived under bridges or at the Salvation Army hostel. Bob was black. He never identified with any risk group for AIDS. The afternoon before Bob was discharged, his sister offered lodging to him. His caregivers were relieved and pleased.

Less than 24 hours after discharge, the emergency medical service telephoned me. Bob had been found naked and catatonic in the middle of a neighborhood street in front of his sister's home. No one was home. The EMS service transported Bob to the medical center where physicians ruled out drug-induced catalepsy or neurological dysfunction. He remained unresponsive for five days. When he emerged from his catatonic state, he became verbally abusive and combative. In full restraints he refused needle sticks and other invasive procedures. Three days of rage and confusion left Bob exhausted. On my last visit with Bob, he sobbed with a visceral sadness I will never forget. He begged for release and forgiveness. Two hours later, Bob hemorrhaged to death.

Not all cases of AIDS psychosis are as stark as this one. But as the AIDS crisis deepens, chaplains, like other health care personnel, will need to become aware that psychotic breaks can occur. Chaplains may spend more "normal" time with patients with AIDS than physicians and must develop precise assessments. When does the behavior of someone push the boundaries of what is real? What feelings can we as chaplains identify during visits with patients? Is the visit frightening? Is the room tight with tension? Irrational behaviors may result from neurological and progressive diseases, but may also be indications of a treatable psychotic episode if properly noted and referred.

The Chaplain's Prophetic Role

Chaplains may not evade the prophetic role into which the biblical mandate thrusts us. Blind institutionalism must be challenged. The catastrophic consequences of progressive HIV disease must be met with compassion and love, and when that

response is absent, chaplains must serve as advocates for people
with AIDS. We must return to the biblical mandate in Isa. 61:1-
3:

> The Spirit of the Lord GOD is upon me,
>   because the LORD has anointed me
> to bring good tidings to the afflicted;
>   he has sent me to bind up the brokenhearted,
> to proclaim liberty to the captives,
>   and the opening of the prison to those who are bound;
> to proclaim the year of the LORD's favor,
>   and the day of vengeance of our God;
>   to comfort all who mourn;
> to grant to those who mourn in Zion—
>   to give them a garland instead of ashes,
> the oil of gladness instead of mourning,
>   the mantle of praise instead of a faint spirit;
> that they may be called oaks of righteousness,
>   the planting of the LORD, that he may be glorified.
> (Parallels can be found in Matt. 11:5; Luke 4:16-20;
>   7:22.)

Ministry to people living with AIDS carries with it a deep
burden of sorrow and grief. The suffering of patients weighs on
the caregivers. Is it possible to heal such brokenheartedness, such
sorrow? Our answer must be "yes." Every untried intervention
offering the hope of restoration to wholeness is worth doing. We
tend to draw back from risk taking. We do not like to be known
as beginners or novices. Thomas Merton said it best, "We do
not want to be beginners. But let us be convinced of the fact that
we will never be anything else but beginners all our lives."[1]

Our path toward healing began by looking at a common element
missing from the problems identified above: community. No real
community exists amidst impersonal institutions that attend to
structures rather than to the people who suffer. No community
exists where desperation, displacement, and disequilibrium are
routine. People with AIDS are stripped of community. We reduce
them to marginal status. When they band together for safety and
a measure of comfort, they join one another in their sameness,
thereby forming yet another social enclave. We do not rock the
boat because their isolation keeps us safe from them.

Community is built on diversity. The apostle Paul said, "There are many members, . . . and one body" (1 Cor. 12:12-26). Paul reminds us that it is those weaker parts that are indispensable, and that in those parts we think less honorable, we invest the greater honor. We are learning from ministry to people with AIDS to invest greater honor in their struggle toward community.

Scott Peck gives us a model for creating community in his book *A Different Drum*. He states that we must begin by identifying our pseudocommunities—those groups of people that form instantly based upon politeness and sameness. Real community takes time, commitment, and sacrifice. Next, we work through the chaos of encountering diversity. We do not run away from it. Once we have worked through the chaos, we can rid ourselves of the need to change, fix, or rescue those who are different from us. We begin to drop our prejudices. Then, says Peck, community begins.[2]

In San Antonio, healing has begun. We are looking at an old problem in a new light. A fledgling community of diverse people is in the making. The Episcopal Diocese of West Texas has offered sanctuary to people with AIDS and a resource for people involved with them. Other parishes are joining us. Laity are graduating from care partner classes and bonding with AIDS patients who need guidance, healing, and reconciliation. We will win. We will lose. We will take risks. God willing, we will learn to love each other.

Notes

1. Thomas Merton, *Contemplative Prayer* (Garden City, N.Y.: Doubleday, 1971), 37.

2. M. Scott Peck, *A Different Drum: Community Making & Peace* (New York: Simon & Schuster, 1987).

Contributors

HERBERT ANDERSON is professor of pastoral theology at the Catholic Theological Union in Chicago.

LAWRENCE E. HOLST is senior vice president, pastoral services, Lutheran General Hospital, Park Ridge, Illinois.

RONALD H. SUNDERLAND is executive director of Equipping Laypeople for Ministry, Houston, Texas.

VIRGIL FRY is a chaplain at the University of Texas M. D. Anderson Cancer Center, Houston, Texas.

NATHAN HUANG is a chaplain at the University of Texas M. D. Anderson Cancer Center, Houston, Texas.

GERI OPSAHL is a seminary student at Lutheran Theological Seminary, Gettysburg, Pennsylvania.

SISTER MARGARET WHOOLEY is a chaplain at the University of Texas M. D. Anderson Cancer Center, Houston, Texas.

BETTY ADAM is assistant to the rector, the Church of St. John the Divine, and adjunct assistant professor, University of St. Thomas, Houston, Texas.

LORNA JEAN T. MILLER is a chaplain, Harris County Hospital District, Houston, Texas.

MARY GRACE is a chaplain currently on sabbatical and preparing a book on the failure of systems in dealing with persons living with AIDS.